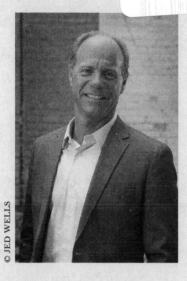

© JED WELLS

Jeff Benedict is the bestselling author of seventeen nonfiction books. He's also a film and television producer. He is the coauthor of the #1 *New York Times* bestseller *Tiger Woods.* The book was the basis of the Emmy-nominated HBO documentary *Tiger,* which Benedict executive produced. *The Dynasty,* the definitive inside story of the New England Patriots under Robert Kraft, Bill Belichick, and Tom Brady, was a *New York Times* bestseller. The book is the basis of a forthcoming 10-part documentary series for Apple TV+, which Benedict is executive producing. His critically acclaimed book *Poisoned* is the basis of a Netflix documentary, which Benedict executive produced. His legal thriller *Little Pink House* was adapted into a motion picture starring Catherine Keener and Jeanne Tripplehorn. Benedict wrote Steve Young's *New York Times* bestselling autobiography *QB,* which was the basis of an *NFL Films* documentary. Benedict's upcoming biography of LeBron James will be published in 2023.

POISONED

The True Story of the Deadly *E. Coli* Outbreak
That Changed the Way Americans Eat

Jeff Benedict

AVID READER PRESS

New York   London   Toronto   Sydney   New Delhi

To Lauren, a daughter whose time was cut short.
And to Roni, a mother who made the right decision.

———

AVID READER PRESS
An Imprint of Simon & Schuster, Inc.
1230 Avenue of the Americas
New York, NY 10020

This Avid Reader Press trade paperback edition January 2023

AVID READER PRESS and colophon are trademarks of Simon & Schuster, Inc.

For information about special discounts for bulk purchases, please contact Simon &
Schuster Special Sales at 1-866-506-1949 or business@simonandschuster.com.

The Simon & Schuster Speakers Bureau can bring authors to your live event.
For more information or to book an event contact the Simon & Schuster Speakers
Bureau at 1-866-248-3049 or visit our website at www.simonspeakers.com.

Interior design by Sarah Pulsford

Manufactured in the United States of America

1   3   5   7   9   10   8   6   4   2

Library of Congress Cataloging-in-Publication Data has been applied for.

ISBN 978-1-9821-9017-0
ISBN 978-1-9821-9018-7 (ebook)

CONTENTS

AUTHOR'S NOTE

Twenty years ago today—on January 17, 1993—the State of Washington's department of health announced that an *E. coli* outbreak was under way in the state and was likely linked to tainted, undercooked hamburgers served at a number of Jack in the Box restaurants. At the time, most Americans had never heard the term *E. coli* O157:H7. The Centers for Disease Control and Prevention (CDC) didn't list it as a reportable disease. Only four state health departments even tracked the pathogen. Other than a few microbiologists and food scientists virtually no one knew the organism existed in food.

But all of that changed as the outbreak rapidly spread throughout the West, tracked by the nightly news at all three major television networks, as well as virtually every big newspaper in the country. The idea that a hamburger could be lethal was a frightening wake-up call. Before the dust settled, over 750 children were poisoned and four had died. Secretary of Agriculture Michael Espy was blindsided. So were the U.S. Department of Agriculture (USDA), the Food and Drug Administration (FDA), and the CDC.

Poisoned is a behind-the-scenes account of the outbreak that introduced America to *E. coli* and opened our eyes to the fact that food safety can be a matter of life and death. It is a jarringly candid version told through the principals at the center of the fast-moving disaster—the families whose children were poisoned, the Jack in the Box executives who were at the helm during the outbreak, the physicians and scientists who identified *E. coli* as the culprit, the lawyers who brought a massive class-action suit against Jack in the Box, and the lawyers who defended the fast-food chain. All of these parties cooperated with me for this book.

I conducted more than two hundred on-the-record interviews. I also received more than a hundred written answers to factual queries sent to sources via email. Most of these electronic communications

involved detailed follow-up questions to prior interviews. I had access
to deposition transcripts, thousands of pages of discovery documents
(internal corporate records from Jack in the Box, medical records from
numerous hospitals and doctors' offices, and insurance records), and
billing records and internal memos from numerous law firms involved
in the Jack in the Box litigation. I was also given access to a trove
of private papers, letters, photographs, and videos associated with the
outbreak.

My primary objective is to tell this epic story in a manner that is
true to the compelling characters who shaped this historic case. I am
indebted to the victims and the survivors who were willing to endure
some emotionally grueling interviews that were often interrupted by
tears, both theirs and mine. I'm thankful to the doctors and lawyers
who took so much time to educate me on the complex medical and legal
issues at play in this case. And without the trust and cooperation of the
Jack in the Box officials, this story would have been incomplete.

The Jack in the Box outbreak is considered the meat industry's
9/11. As soon as hamburgers killed kids, everything changed. Congressional hearings were held. The national media put a spotlight on the
industry. State and federal health codes were upgraded. *E. coli* became
a reportable disease among all state health departments. Mandatory
internal cooking temperatures for beef were raised to 165 degrees
throughout the country. Even the warning labels that you see on all the
meat and poultry sold in the supermarket today are a direct result of
the Jack in the Box outbreak.

But the Jack in the Box case has had implications that reach far beyond
the meat industry. The case gave rise to the nation's first and only law
firm dedicated solely to representing victims of food poisoning. Based
in Seattle, Marler Clark LLP is the creation of Bill Marler, who as a
fledgling personal-injury lawyer took on Jack in the Box and in the
process became convinced that the problem of food safety extended far
beyond one restaurant chain and one pathogen. His firm, which works
with physicians, former public-health officials, and scientists around the
world, has helped transform the way outbreaks are handled by health
officials, insurance companies, and the news media. Marler has also led

the charge on food-safety reform in Washington. Without question, few individuals have had more influence on the shape and direction of food-safety policy in the U.S. over the past twenty years.

Another far-reaching legacy of the Jack in the Box case is the area of public awareness. In the outbreak's aftermath, books like *Fast Food Nation* and *The Omnivore's Dilemma* became runaway best sellers. Farmer's markets sprang up everywhere. The organic movement exploded. Grocery chains like Trader Joe's and Whole Foods have become billion-dollar companies by marketing natural and wholesome foods. Today even Wal-Mart offers a large selection of organic products.

In short, since 1993, food safety has emerged as a serious public-health issue in America. The CDC estimates that foodborne disease causes about 48 million illnesses per year. Roughly one in six Americans get sick from bad food. Many of these cases are mild gastroenteritis, commonly referred to as the stomach bug. But too many food poisoning cases are more serious, resulting in approximately 125,000 hospitalizations and 3,000 deaths annually. The fatalities are often children and the elderly.

Besides the obvious human toll, there's an economic side to this. Foodborne illness in the United States costs about $152 billion a year. That's the sum of medical expenses, insurance costs, and lost wages. It's a staggering number. But it's not surprising given the number of major outbreaks in recent years. In 2010, more than half a billion eggs were recalled after nearly two thousand people became ill with *Salmonella* poisoning. A year before that, nine people died in a *Salmonella* outbreak linked to a peanut-manufacturing plant. Hundreds of food products from breakfast cereal to energy bars had to be recalled, costing food manufacturers over a billion dollars.

E. coli O157:H7 is often more deadly than *Salmonella*. Although beef remains the most common vector of *E. coli* poisoning, the list of other foods responsible for major *E. coli* outbreaks is bewildering: spinach, unpasteurized apple juice, peppers, bagged lettuce, sprouts, raw milk, cilantro, and cheese, to name just a few. *E. coli* even found its way into raw cookie dough in 2009.

There has been some good news. On January 4, 2011, President Barack Obama signed the FDA Food Safety Modernization Act (FSMA), the most sweeping reform of our food-safety laws in more than seventy years. It shifted the focus from responding to contamination to preventing it. The bad news is that Congress and the Obama administration have failed to fund the law. Meantime, in September 2011, the U.S. was hit with its deadliest food poison outbreak in one hundred years when thirty-three people died after eating *Listeria*-contaminated cantaloupes.

There are now more than two hundred known diseases transmitted through food. The Jack in the Box outbreak is a cautionary tale that points out the significance of food safety. It's also an inspiring tale of courage and resourcefulness. Despite the terrible human loss associated with this case, a remarkable number of things were done right in the aftermath. It's a story that will forever change the way you look at what you eat.

Jeff Benedict
January 21, 2013
Buena Vista, Virginia

CAST OF CHARACTERS

The Principals

William "Bill" Marler
Attorney who sued Jack in the Box on behalf of poisoned children

Brianne Kiner
Nine-year-old *E. coli* victim

Suzanne Kiner
Mother of Brianne Kiner

Robert Nugent
President of Jack in the Box

David Theno
VP of product safety for Jack in the Box

Bob Piper
Attorney for Jack in the Box

Denis Stearns
Attorney for Jack in the Box

Key Players
In order of their appearance

Lauren Rudolph
The first child to die in the Jack in the Box outbreak

Roni Austin
Lauren Rudolph's mother

Dr. Glen Billman
Associate Director of Pathology at Children's Hospital–San Diego

Julie Marler
Wife of attorney William Marler

Dr. Phil Tarr
Head of Gastroenterology at Seattle Children's Hospital

John Kobayashi
Washington State epidemiologist

Ken Dunkley
VP of quality assurance for Jack in the Box

Jack Goodall
CEO of Foodmaker, Inc., parent company of Jack in the Box

Jody Powell
Advisor to Bob Nugent during congressional hearings on *E. coli*

Dr. Richard Siegler
Nephrologist specializing in *E. coli* infection at University of
Utah Hospital

Fred Gordon
Attorney for Jack in the Box

Bruce Clark
Attorney for Jack in the Box

Lynn Sarko
Managing partner at Keller Rohrback, the law firm that filed a class-action suit against Jack in the Box

Mark Griffin
Class-action attorney at Keller Rohrback

Chris Pence
Co-counsel with Keller Rohrback in class-action case

Mike Canaan
Private investigator hired by the Kiner family

Judge Terry Carroll
Special master in the class-action case against Jack in the Box

Brad Keller
Attorney who represented Bill Marler in the dispute with Keller Rohrback

George Kargianis
Personal-injury attorney who partnered with Bill Marler

Simeon Osborn
Personal-injury attorney who partnered with Bill Marler

Mike Watkins
Personal-injury attorney who partnered with Bill Marler

Judge Lawrence Irving
Mediator in the Brianne Kiner settlement

A NOTE TO READERS

This is an account of the most seminal foodborne illness outbreak of the past fifty years. Law, medicine, politics, and business shape the story. But at its core, this story is about ordinary people swept up in an extraordinary tragedy.

I chose to tell this story through the voices of the people who lived it, while staying true to the memory of those who died. Almost all dialogue is recounted in real time, meaning as it happened. There are some instances, however, where I put quotes around a statement that someone said to me. In those instances, I use the verb explained.

I have also attributed unspoken thoughts, feelings, and conclusions to people in the book. Those come from the person him- or herself or, in a few instances, from a person who had direct knowledge of the other person's views.

POISONED

1

SILENT NIGHT

Thursday, December 24, 1992
San Diego, California

RONI KNEW SOMETHING WAS WRONG WHEN SHE FOUND BLOOD IN THE toilet after her six-year-old daughter, Lauren Rudolph, slid off the seat. By the time Roni and her husband, Dick, got Lauren to Children's Hospital, she was doubled over and moaning. Her diarrhea had become so fast and furious that her parents had outfitted her in a big makeshift diaper. Lauren's pediatrician had called ahead and arranged for a physician to meet them in the ER. "We've got one very sick little girl," the doctor said in a reassuring voice as soon as he laid eyes on Lauren. He took Lauren from Roni and cradled her in his arms. "We'll take care of her."

Roni and Dick spent the rest of the day waiting and wondering what was going on. Lauren had always been an active, healthy child. A couple of days earlier Roni had kept her home from school on account of a slight fever, stomach cramps, and the runs. It looked like typical flu symptoms until blood showed up in the diarrhea and all of a sudden Lauren was too weak to walk on her own. Roni and Dick felt fine, as did their eleven-year-old son, Michael. Whatever Lauren had didn't seem to be affecting the rest of the family.

By morning Lauren was transferred to the ICU (Intensive Care Unit) and given powerful painkillers. The doctors felt there was a good chance that Lauren's appendix had failed. The small organ attaches to the large intestine and has the job of destroying microorganisms that carry diseases and enter the body through the digestive tract. That, doctors said, might explain the bloody diarrhea. In the morning, Lauren would receive a barium test to determine whether an appendectomy were necessary. Until then, she needed a sound night's sleep. The medication would assure that.

"You can stay overnight with her if you want to," the lead doctor told the Rudolphs, and assured them that Lauren would be out until morning.

Roni and Dick looked at each other. They were thinking the same thing. It was late on Christmas Eve. Their eleven-year-old son had

Six-year-old Lauren Rudolph shortly before being hospitalized with a stomach illness.

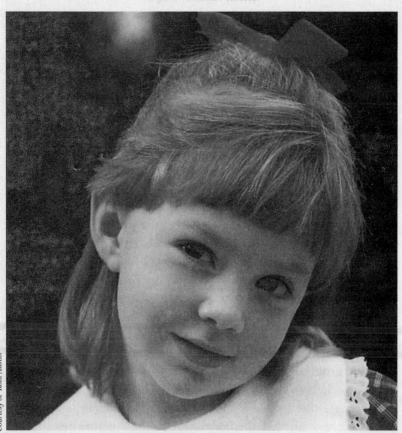

been waiting at a neighbor's house all day, worried about his sister. With Lauren sedated, they decided to go home, reassure their son, and gather up some Christmas presents to bring back to the hospital for Lauren to open in the morning. They told the doctors they'd be back before 7:00 a.m.

That night, before getting into bed, Roni went into Lauren's bedroom. She felt lonely seeing her daughter's empty bed. She sat down on it, thinking it didn't seem like Christmas Eve. Out of the corner of her eye she spotted a handwritten note on the floor beside the bed. She leaned over and picked it up.

> *Dear Santa,*
> *I don't feel so good. Please make me*
> *better for Christmas.*
>
> *Lauren*

Roni's eyes welled up. It was after midnight. She had to get some sleep.

When Lauren awoke the next morning her family was there with presents. Roni handed her a gift-wrapped box. It contained a beautiful Christmas dress with jewels on it. Lauren loved pretty clothes. She smiled and said she couldn't wait to wear it. But she was too weak to open anything else. So Michael read her stories and fed her ice chips. It was afternoon when the results of the barium test came back— negative. Lauren did not have appendicitis.

Now what?

More tests, the doctors said.

New tubes and lines were connected to Lauren's body, but her condition only worsened as the day wore on. She never got around to opening her other Christmas presents. She kept complaining of unquenchable thirst. Other than occasional ice chips, all her fluids were being administered through an IV.

On the morning of the 26th Roni arrived back at the hospital with her son. Dick was in the room with Lauren, leaning over her bed, gripping her little hands. When Roni saw Dick's eyes, she noticed they were red. She could tell he'd been crying. But Dick never cried. He had served in the napalm infantry during the Vietnam War, where he had seen unimaginable horrors. Since then he just didn't cry.

A chill ran through Roni. It scared her to see Dick that way. She reached for his hand and he nodded for her to follow him to the doorway.

"What happened?" Roni whispered.

"Lauren said she is going to die," he said softly. "She just knows she is going to die."

Roni looked back into the room at Lauren, tossing and turning in discomfort while a nurse attended to her. Dick asked where Michael was. Roni had left him in the ICU waiting area. Dick decided to take him out for breakfast; he shouldn't see his sister this way. Roni headed back into the room to sit with Lauren. She pulled up a chair beside the bed, took Lauren's little hand, and hugged her. "It's going to be okay, Lauren," she whispered. "It's going to be okay."

"Is the doctor going to make me better?"

That got her nurse's attention. She flashed Roni a tortured smile.

Roni had always viewed herself as a fixer. But she had an awful sense of helplessness. "Yes, you're going to get better," Roni said, starting to stroke Lauren's feet. "You are in the hospital. Things are going to be okay."

"Okay," Lauren said, crying and closing her eyes.

"I'm so, so sorry, Lauren," Roni said, continuing to massage her feet. "I'm so, so sorry."

Roni had been married to Dick for thirteen years before she had Michael at age thirty-four. She was thirty-nine when she had Lauren. By then Roni was an established interior designer, and she didn't want to give up her career. But she refused to put her children in day care, figuring she'd waited a long time to have them, so she wanted to be with them. She told her friends she wasn't about to pawn her kids off on someone else for child rearing. Instead, Roni juggled motherhood with a full-time job. Confident, driven, and meticulously organized, Roni was in good shape, too. At forty-four she could still turn a man's head.

But her best asset was her attitude. It reflected the San Diego weather—always sunny. She just believed there wasn't anything she couldn't do. When Lauren enrolled in preschool, Roni volunteered there as a teacher's aide twice a week. In the afternoons, she'd take Lauren to work with her, teaching her about design, color schemes, floral arrangements, and fashion. Somehow Roni still managed to get dinner on the table each night.

The only thing she didn't have time for was reflection. Life was too fast for that. Lauren's illness had put the brakes on everything, though. Sitting around the hospital for a few days had Roni thinking about a lot of things, most of which traced back to her family and their time together. She just refused to believe that Lauren's illness—whatever it was—was anything more than a temporary interruption. They were in a great hospital with top doctors, she kept telling herself. Surely they'd get to the bottom of this. The situation would turn around. It had to.

Suddenly it dawned on Roni that she was alone in the room with Lauren. The nurses were gone. Unaccustomed to sitting still so long, she'd lost track of time. But her hand was still caressing Lauren's foot. She looked up at Lauren and noticed her lips were blue.

"Oh my God!" she shouted to no one.

She called Lauren's name. But she didn't appear to be breathing.

"Oh my God," she screamed, turning toward the doorway. "SOMEBODY HELP ME! SOMEBODY HELP ME NOW!"

Two nurses rushed in, trailed by a doctor. "Get the mother out of here," he ordered as he struggled to revive Lauren.

"I'm not going anyplace!" Roni yelled, crying hysterically as two more medical personnel pushed past her.

"Yes, you are," the doctor shouted. "Take her out."

"No, no, that's my baby," she cried as the nurses hooked their arms under Roni's and guided her outside, assuring her it was for the best. An alarm was going off. So was a beeper. It seemed like more and more people in medical uniforms were rushing into Lauren's room.

It was a couple of hours before a senior physician came out to meet with Roni and Dick. The doctor took Roni's hand. "We got her heart started again," he began. Roni took a deep breath. "But," the doctor continued softly, "Lauren had a heart attack. We've got her stabilized and—"

"How can a healthy six-year-old have a heart attack?" Roni interrupted.

The doctor provided a short medical explanation, something about blood flow. It didn't make sense to Roni. Kids aren't supposed to suffer heart attacks.

"What's going to happen?" Roni said.

"Is she going to be okay?" Dick chimed in.

The doctor said that Lauren was in a medically induced coma.

The word *coma* stunned Roni and Dick.

The doctor explained that when a patient goes into cardiac arrest and there's a neurological insult, the brain starts swelling, which is very dangerous. A drug-induced coma prevents seizures and enables the body to conserve much-needed energy. Lauren's kidneys had failed. Other vital organs were at risk. The coma offered the best chance for her vital organs to regain strength. "The next twenty-four hours are critical," he said.

More than a day passed without any changes. Roni and Dick wanted answers. At this point they still didn't know what was wreaking all this havoc in their daughter's body.

A doctor took them into a private consultation room off of the ICU. "She should have come out of the coma by now," he said. "But she hasn't."

Roni wanted to know why.

"The heart attacks created such havoc that she . . ." His voice trailed off.

"That she what?" Roni said.

The doctor explained that the damage to Lauren's brain was irreversible.

Roni exhaled and closed her eyes. Dick said nothing.

"So what does all this mean?" Roni asked.

"If we take her off life support, most likely she will not be able to breathe on her own."

Dick wanted to know Lauren's chances for survival.

"We need you to be honest," Roni said.

The doctor's expression told them everything they needed to know. Her prospects were grave. Blood supply to Lauren's brain had been compromised. If, by chance, she did survive, she wouldn't be the child she had been before getting ill. Her vital organs, particularly the brain, had sustained serious damage. "We can keep her on a life-support system," he said. "I'll give you some time."

Numb, Roni and Dick just looked at each other. Death had come so swiftly. There hadn't even been time to pray. They didn't need to discuss anything. Maybe it was their state of mind, the shock. Maybe it was the doctor's convincing case, so clinical and clear. Whatever the reason, they were on the same page. The damage to her heart and brain were irreversible. Lauren would probably never run or play again. There was a good chance she would never be lucid. They couldn't put her or the family through that.

When Roni and Dick returned to Lauren's room, the sight of her only confirmed their decision. She looked yellow and lifeless. She was unrecognizable as the girl in the picture of her that hung above her bed. The picture showed a smiling girl with short bangs in the front and long hair in the back. She was missing a couple of baby teeth. She had her whole life in front of her. But not anymore. And the doctors couldn't explain why. Their best guess was that Lauren had succumbed to a particularly virulent strain of flu. It didn't make sense to Roni. Nothing did.

Roni told the doctor they had decided to have the life-support system disconnected.

"Is there anything you want to do first?" the doctor said respectfully.

"Well, one thing I promised Lauren that I'd do before Christmas was put fingernail polish on her toes," she said, wiping away tears. "That's what she wanted. You know, she was a girl's girl."

"Wait here," the doctor said.

A few minutes later a nurse entered the room. "What color did she want them painted?" the nurse asked.

"Bright pink," Roni said.

The nurse nodded and smiled.

"Oh God, I'm a mess," Roni said.

The nurse returned fifteen minutes later and handed Roni a bottle of pink nail polish.

Time seemed to stop as Roni artfully dabbed each tiny nail. She'd never done anything so deliberately before. While she waited for the polish to dry, Roni held Lauren and sang a lullaby she had sung to her as a baby:

> *Mama's baby.*
> *Mama's baby.*
> *Mama's baby.*
> *Mama's baby girl.*

When the time came to remove Lauren's ventilator, Dick squeezed his daughter's limp hands while Roni pressed the child against her heart, clutching her until she felt the last breath go out of her.

"We'll never be the same again," Dick said, weeping. "We'll never be the same."

Melting in tears, Roni just sat there holding Lauren. Five days earlier she had stayed home from school with a stomach ache. Now she was gone.

As the Associate Director of Pathology at Children's Hospital– San Diego, Dr. Glen Billman ran the morgue. At thirty-six he had performed more than three hundred autopsies on children. Normally when a child dies in a hospital, the cause of death is readily apparent. But even before Billman laid eyes on Lauren Rudolph, he was mystified by her medical record. It indicated she had gone into cardiac arrest just two days after being admitted. She was resuscitated, but not before blood flow to the brain had ceased, resulting in cerebral edema. The thing Billman couldn't get over was the speed of Lauren's decline. Yet there was nothing in her medical history to explain heart problems.

A six-year-old with no chronic illness has gone from perfectly healthy to dead in six days? He couldn't explain that.

Medical mysteries like this were what had prompted Billman to become a pathologist. He had a natural inclination toward solving riddles, a talent he used on behalf of grieving parents desperate for answers.

Reading through Lauren's record, he came to "Diagnostic Considerations." The attending physician had listed as a possible cause hemolytic-uremic syndrome (HUS), a rare disease that attacks red blood cells, leading to anemia and kidney failure. That intrigued Billman. He had just read some new medical research identifying *E. coli* as the primary cause of HUS.

Billman knew *E. coli* to be an abbreviation for *Escherichia coli*, a tube-shaped bacterium named after the German bacteriologist who identified it as an organism found in the stomachs of warm-blooded animals, particularly cattle. Most strains of *E. coli* are harmless to humans. But one strain—*E. coli* O157:H7 can be deadly. Microbiologists had recently identified undercooked ground beef as the primary vector of the deadly *E. coli* strain. But Billman had never autopsied someone who had died of HUS from *E. coli* O157:H7. He called upstairs to the infectious-disease lab and requested fungal and bacterial cultures on Lauren.

Then he opened Lauren's abdomen. The size of her bowel stunned him. It should have been an inch and a half in diameter. It was more than twice that size. It felt soft and boggy when Billman pushed on it with his index finger. A healthy bowel is firm and pink with a vascular arcade of blood vessels visible in the transparent surface. Lauren's was the color of swamp water.

The inner wall of the colon revealed obvious signs of hemorrhaging consistent with clot formation in the blood vessels. Lauren's kidneys showed the same scenario—sheared red blood cells leading to clot formation leading to the obstruction of blood flow in the kidney. The medical literature indicated that *E. coli* O157:H7 manufactures a toxin that attacks red blood cells, ultimately destroying the scaffolding of the blood vessels, essentially cutting off blood flow to the vital organs.

Under a microscope, Billman could see the invasion of bacteria in the colon wall. The capillaries were filled with clots, leaving a dead zone that looked like a black band of hemorrhage and clots. "I've never seen anything like this before," Billman said to one of his colleagues. "To go from a completely healthy child to a child with this pathology is unheard-of."

Then Billman got the stool cultures back from the lab. They confirmed the presence of *E. coli* O157:H7. As soon as Billman finished his examination he called upstairs to the Infectious Disease Unit and notified them that a previously normal, healthy child had died of HUS brought on by *E. coli* poisoning. Then he reached out to the San Diego Department of Public Health. Billman had no idea where Lauren Rudolph had come in contact with *E. coli*. But he was no believer in random chance. Odds were that a deadly bug was on the loose.

"In hundreds of autopsies I've never seen anything like this," he explained. "When something really unusual happens, you need to be worried that something really unusual might be going on."

Despite the urgency of Billman's tone, his message fell on deaf ears. The health department had no other reported cases of *E. coli* poisoning. Billman wasn't surprised, given that *E. coli* was not yet on the list of reportable infectious diseases in California. That meant physicians and hospitals weren't required to report it. Billman was looking for the county to take some proactive steps to notify health care officials that something might be afoot.

Instead, the health department chose a wait-and-see approach.

———

San Diego attorney Rick Waite had just returned with his family from a holiday trip to the East Coast. There was a message from Roni Austin on the Waites' home answering machine. Waite's six-year-old daughter, Katherine, was Lauren's best friend. Undoubtedly, Waite figured, Roni had called in hopes of getting the girls together over the Christmas break. They were, after all, pretty inseparable. As soon as he finished unpacking, Waite called Roni at home.

"Lauren's dead," she told him.

Those two words froze Waite. The news was impossible to fathom.

Blow by blow, Roni related the tragic events of the previous five days.

The longer he listened, the more befuddled Waite became. A little over a week earlier, Katherine had been with Lauren, who certainly had appeared to be perfectly healthy. What could account for such a rapid decline in health?

Roni had no answer. She couldn't explain it. No one could. That's what was driving her mad. All she knew was that Lauren's funeral was a couple of days away.

Waite assured her that he and his family would be there. And he pledged to support Roni in any way she needed.

Planning the funeral of her only daughter was something Roni had never anticipated. After a final meeting with the funeral home, she returned to her house, where she retrieved a message from a woman at the San Diego Department of Public Health. "I'm very busy trying to close your daughter's medical case," the message said. "My time is premium and I would appreciate you getting back to me at the earliest time you have available." The caller repeated her name and number.

Seething at the callousness of the woman's tone, Roni immediately called the woman back.

Without a word about Lauren, the health official started right in. "I just have a few quick questions in order to close this case," she said. "Did your daughter ever clean the cat box?"

"What?"

The woman repeated the question. Roni informed her they didn't own a cat.

Next the woman asked if Lauren had eaten at any fast-food restaurants the week before she got sick.

"I don't know," Roni shouted. "What does that have to do with anything? My daughter is dead!"

The health official paused before explaining why she was asking where Lauren had eaten. Then she repeated the question.

"My husband had taken Lauren to McDonald's or Wendy's or Jack in the Box. But I don't know which one. I would have to ask him. I still don't know what this has to do with anything. My daughter is dead."

When Rick Waite filed into Solana Beach Presbyterian Church for Lauren Rudolph's funeral, the forty-one-year-old father struggled to keep his emotions in check as he laid eyes on the coffin at the head of the chapel. It was so . . . small.

White satin lined the coffin. Lauren had on her Christmas dress, the one she never had the opportunity to wear in life. Her father's

Purple Heart was pinned to her collar. Roni's wedding dress was next to her.

Fittingly, the service included a series of Christmas carols. But when the organist began playing "Silent Night," Waite broke down, his eyes shifting back and forth between the still coffin and Roni, trembling.

> *Silent night, holy night*
> *All is calm, all is bright*
> *Round yon Virgin Mother and Child*
> *Holy Infant so tender and mild*
> *Sleep in heavenly peace*
> *Sleep in heavenly peace*

Waite had always loved to sing "Silent Night." It was his favorite carol. But he knew he'd never sing that carol again. It would always remind him of Lauren Rudolph in a tiny coffin at the head of the church.

The next night, Waite got another call from Roni. She told him about the bizarre call she'd received from the health department.

"Something is going on," Waite said. "And something is not right."

Roni felt the same way.

"I think you should get an attorney to represent you and to help you find out what happened to Lauren," Waite said.

"I'd like you to be my lawyer," she said.

"Roni, that's not my field," he said, explaining that she needed a personal-injury lawyer. "I'm a business lawyer and a real estate guy."

"No, I want you to help me," she insisted.

He tried again to dissuade her, telling her she'd be better served by retaining someone who specialized in wrongful-death cases.

Under the circumstances, Roni wanted a lawyer she trusted. And she strongly preferred a lawyer with young children. Waite fit the bill perfectly. Her goal, Roni explained, was to get to the bottom of what had killed Lauren.

Waite agreed to help. But he had no idea what he was dealing with. Neither did the public-health officials in San Diego.

2

CHOMPING AT THE BIT

Tuesday, January 5, 1993
Seattle, Washington

TRYING NOT TO WAKE HIS WIFE AND ONE-YEAR-OLD DAUGHTER, MORGAN, in the adjoining bedroom, thirty-three-year-old Bill Marler quietly toweled off before hurriedly using his fingers to straighten his freshly clipped hair. He shaved, setting off his chiseled face and recessed green eyes. Then he threw on a suit and tie before glancing in the mirror. The young lawyer liked what he saw. Even in business attire, his 5'10", 165-pound frame looked muscular and trim.

Yet Bill was frustrated as he ducked out the front door of his modest one-bedroom cabin situated on the edge of an Indian reservation near Bainbridge Island. A cold morning wind came off Puget Sound as he fired up the engine on his 1963 Chevy pickup before scraping a thin layer of frost from the windshield. All he could think about was the date: January 5, 1993. It had been highlighted on his calendar for months as the day Washington State would carry out its first execution since 1963. Serial child molester Westley Allan Dodd had been sentenced to death for the murders of ten-year-old William Neer and his eleven-year-old brother, Cole. Dodd had also confessed to raping and strangling four-year-old Lee Iseli.

The Neer and Iseli families had been Bill's clients. But he didn't represent them anymore. That's why he was so frustrated. After Bill had spent a year building an airtight case against the State of Washington for negligently allowing Dodd—a serial child rapist—to be out on the street at the time when he encountered the Neer and Iseli children, the state agreed to pay the families seven-figure settlements. But before the settlement was reached, Bill's law firm, Keller Rohrback, forced him to withdraw from the case and turn it over to another firm. The problem was that Keller Rohrback was one of the premier insurance-defense firms in Seattle, and most of its clients were corporations, insurance companies, and government entities, including the State of Washington. At the last minute, the firm decided that it didn't make sense to sue the state in one matter and defend it in other ones. Bill didn't see a conflict—the other suits had all been resolved and they involved different state agencies. But as a third-year associate, he had no say in the matter.

That fact that all those legal fees ended up going to another lawyer wasn't what roiled Bill. It was the idea that the first high-profile case of his career—one that put a spotlight on an important public safety issue, namely the need to protect children from pedophiles—had been taken out from under him. Bill had joined Keller Rohrback under the

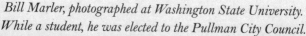

Bill Marler, photographed at Washington State University.
While a student, he was elected to the Pullman City Council.

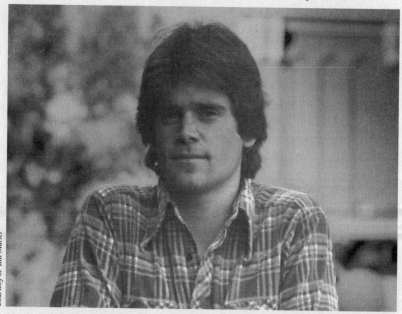

pretense that he'd be free to build up a personal-injury practice. After toiling away for three years on slip-and-fall cases and automobile accidents, he'd finally landed some clients that gave him a sense of purpose beyond generating legal fees. He tried innovative things, like interviewing Dodd on death row and getting him to make a confession that implicated the state. His groundbreaking suit was featured in the *Seattle Times*, enabling Bill to start to make a name for himself. None of that mattered now.

He hopped behind the wheel and drove his pickup to the Bainbridge Island ferry terminal. A part of him felt like taking a detour and heading to the state penitentiary in Walla Walla to witness the execution. Despite opposing the death penalty, he still felt a loyalty to his former clients. But instead, he parked in the commuter lot and boarded the ferry for another routine morning commute to Seattle. Not in the mood for company, he found a seat away from everyone else. Blankly staring out the rain-splattered windows of the ferry, Bill retraced the steps that had brought him to this point.

During Bill's junior year of high school the local sheriff in his hometown had ticketed him for flashing his high beams. All of Bill's buddies feared this guy, known for harassing teenagers. Fed up, Bill looked up the traffic code, and he got the sheriff to admit in court that he had flashed Bill first. The point was self-evident: if Bill had broken the law, so had the sheriff. The judge grinned, issued Bill a verbal warning, and dismissed the ticket. Afterward the local prosecutor wanted a word with Bill. "Son, you should go to law school," he said, patting Bill on the shoulder. From that moment on, Bill had never thought seriously about doing anything else.

Yet his path from high school to law school was an unlikely one. Before college he spent a summer working as a migrant farm hand. Then, during his sophomore year at Washington State University, Bill ran for a seat on the Pullman City Council. He was only twenty at the time. But over an illegally obtained beer, the student body president convinced him that with so many students living in the city there ought to be a student voice in local government. Bill found it funny that the law considered him old enough to hold public office, yet too young to drink. He borrowed the twelve dollars for the filing fee and announced his candidacy against a woman who had been in office almost as long as Bill had been alive. The incumbent also happened to own the largest department store in the city. She had money, connections, and a take-charge wardrobe. Bill was broke; his only friends were students; and his one suit came from Goodwill. Just before the start of the first debate, the incumbent made sure Bill knew his place. "Bill," she said condescendingly before the microphones were live, "the way you dress is why merchants in this town lose money." Then she continued to talk down to him for the next hour.

Bill shrugged it off. He didn't really expect to win and he knew enough to know he was in way over his head. But it didn't take him long to figure out that politics is really a people business, and Bill was a people person. He campaigned night and day, eventually knocking on virtually every door in his district. The incumbent didn't bother. Bill won by fifty-seven votes, and his face ended up on television and in all the newspapers. He made state history. At twenty he became the youngest person ever elected to public office in Washington.

Just like that, Bill's life got really serious really fast. There was no time for frat parties and plying girls with alcohol in hopes of getting them into bed. He'd been on the front page. People expected him to know city ordinances, tax codes, and zoning regulations, but he didn't. To get up to speed, Bill practically moved into City Hall, spending more time there than in class. That was when he met his first wife.

About six months after taking office, Bill was hanging out in the Planning Department, looking over maps, when a tanned blond in a sexy white dress walked in. She looked too good to belong there. Bill said hello and the woman introduced herself as the new architect that had just been hired by the city's Engineering Department. One thing led to another and before long Bill was a twenty-two-year-old elected official who was a full-time student who was married to an architect.

Life was complicated. Yet Bill liked it that way. By the time he reached law school, at twenty-eight, his life experience gave him a big advantage over his younger classmates. In his first year he landed a part-time job clerking at a big firm in Seattle. Then he secured a coveted clerkship with a superior court judge. He just seemed destined to do great things—until his wife said she wanted a divorce.

The realization that he wasn't everything to his wife made him suddenly question everything about himself. It occurred to him that his workaholic approach to law school might have cost him his marriage. Maybe if his wife had seen a little more of him she wouldn't have been seeing someone else. Bill ended up living alone on a friend's sailboat. Resentment set in, and he went into a year-long funk that cost him a job at one law firm and nearly caused him to forfeit his last year of law school.

Nobody heard more about Bill's marriage crisis than the handful of lawyers he jogged with every day during lunch hour. Every time Bill brought up his wife, they tried to assure him that he'd have other opportunities. But he didn't want other opportunities. He wanted what he had had with his wife: the clever humor, drinks at Pike's Place on Friday nights, the lovemaking, and the common goal of building careers and a family together.

The oldest lawyer in the group was Egil "Bud" Krogh, a key figure in the Nixon administration who served a brief prison term after pleading guilty to federal conspiracy charges in connection with the Watergate scandal. Disbarred in 1975, Krogh had been readmitted to practice law in Washington State in 1980 and had returned to practicing law in Seattle. One afternoon as Krogh and the rest of the group completed their run, they were catching their breath outside the Seattle YMCA when Bill brought up his marital situation again. Krogh had heard enough.

"It's time to stop whining," Krogh said unapologetically. "You don't have it that bad."

That got everyone's attention.

"When I was in prison," Krogh continued, beads of sweat dripping from his forehead, "I had lost everything: job, income, profession, respect, and personal freedom."

Embarrassed, Bill said nothing.

"Your situation is shitty," Krogh said. "But it ain't that bad. Get your shit together, Bill."

Krogh stirred Bill. But he didn't truly bounce back until his divorce was finalized several months later and he began dating Julie Dueck, an attractive receptionist from the firm where he had clerked. Younger and adventuresome, Julie had grown up on Bainbridge Island and loved the outdoors. She had also overcome a life-threatening bout with cancer at nineteen. She was in the final stages of treatment when she started seeing Bill. They got each other through some tough times and did a lot of fishing, boating, and camping together. The first time they made love was on a remote beach near the Canadian border on a crisp Indian summer day in October. Bill had never felt anything like that. Afterward, he clasped his hands behind his head, closed his eyes, and reclined against a large piece of driftwood. "I wish it could be like this forever," he said, facing the sun.

"You know, I do, too," Julie said, reaching for her balled-up sweatshirt on the blanket. She removed a ring from the pocket and handed it to Bill. "That's why I want you to marry me."

Bill had never encountered a woman like Julie before. In 1988 they exchanged vows in a private ceremony. Before long they had their first child together. Meantime, Bill bounced from one firm to another before landing the job at Keller Rohrback, earning fifty thousand dollars per year. The stability and the income were nice. But he was more restless than ever. His law career just wasn't advancing as fast as he had thought it would. More than anything he longed for a sense of purpose—now.

As he exited the ferry in Seattle and trudged up the hill toward the Washington Mutual Bank Building that housed his firm's offices, he couldn't help wondering if he were in the right place.

3

SOMETHING BAD

One Week Later
Tuesday, January 12, 1993

As Gastroenterology junior faculty at Children's Hospital in Seattle and a professor at the medical school, Dr. Phil Tarr had a lot on his plate. And after a long weekend, he had a lot of catching up to do on his first day back. In a white shirt and tie with a beeper clipped to his belt, Tarr grabbed a clipboard and started down the hallway to make his rounds. He immediately bumped into one of his colleagues, a kidney specialist who served as the pediatric unit's nephrologist. When Tarr asked how things had gone on the floor over the weekend, the nephrologist said he'd been unusually busy.

Tarr was surprised.

"Well," the nephrologist said, "I've got a couple of kids in ICU with HUS."

Tarr paused. He was all too familiar with HUS and its deadly potential in children. As the leading pediatric authority in the U.S. on *E. coli* O157:H7, he and his colleagues had produced most of the research supporting the connection between the pathogen and HUS. He knew that since consumption of undercooked ground beef was the primary way humans got *E. coli*, HUS was typically a disease that was more prevalent during barbecue season than in the dead of winter. *This is January*, Tarr thought to himself. *HUS almost never occurs in January.*

Tarr then returned to the clinical office to pick up his messages. Two were marked "urgent." Both were from pediatricians calling with questions about patients with bloody diarrhea. *That's odd*, Tarr thought. He immediately returned the calls, and both pediatricians described patients with the same symptoms: strong abdominal pain, bloody diarrhea, little or no fever. And both children had previously been healthy.

Tarr's instincts were telling him there was an *E. coli* outbreak afoot. However, the time of year was off. Outbreaks are more common in summer months. Nonetheless, the appearance of randomly located cases throughout the region was consistent with a few previous outbreaks he knew about. The two pediatricians Tarr had called were treating patients that lived more than fifty miles apart. The two patients in the ICU didn't live close to each other either.

Sensing trouble, Tarr tracked down Dr. Dennis Christie, who shared responsibility with Tarr for fielding calls from pediatricians facing unusual situations.

"Have you gotten any calls about bloody diarrhea?" Tarr asked him.

Christie had. That morning two pediatricians had called him with similar cases.

Tarr jotted down their names and called them right away. It was more of the same: two children who lived far apart, both with severe bloody

---

Dr. Phil Tarr was considered the leading expert on E. coli *when children started showing up at Children's Hospital in Seattle with symptoms of food poisoning.*

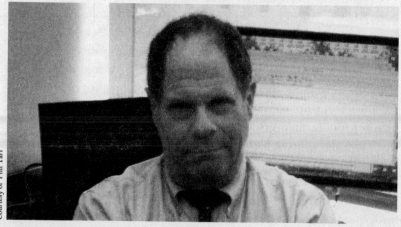

diarrhea. That brought the total number of sick children with these symptoms to six. Scratching his head, Tarr hung up the phone and looked up to discover one of the sharpest residents standing in his office doorway.

The young man could tell from the expression on Tarr's face that something was wrong. "What's going on?" he asked.

"Something is happening out there," Tarr said. "I'm hearing about all these kids with bloody diarrhea."

"Huh, sounds interesting."

"Sounds like *E. coli*," Tarr said.

The resident raised his eyebrows and disappeared without saying another word, leaving Tarr to ponder why six kids in the greater Seattle area had suddenly come down with bloody diarrhea.

Tarr had first gotten interested in bloody diarrhea shortly after graduating from the Yale School of Medicine and accepting an internship in Seattle at Children's Hospital. One of his first patients was a four-year-old boy with HUS that developed after he suffered from bloody diarrhea. Most kids with bloody diarrhea do not develop HUS. In fact, Tarr's four-year-old patient had a sister who also had bloody diarrhea, but she didn't get HUS. That's what intrigued Tarr. There seemed to be no explanation for why some kids with bloody diarrhea got violently ill with HUS and others didn't.

Having already been interested in infectious diseases when he was a student, Tarr started researching HUS cases in Seattle soon after he arrived at Children's. That was when he discovered the preponderance of cases in summer and fall. Tarr wondered why the disease seemed to go quiet during winter and spring. Then he read a report written by a team of physicians and epidemiologists and published in the *New England Journal of Medicine*:

> We investigated two outbreaks of an unusual gastrointestinal illness that affected at least 47 people in Oregon and Michigan in February through March and May through June 1982. The illness was characterized by severe crampy abdominal pain, initially watery diarrhea followed by grossly bloody diarrhea, and little or no fever. It was associated with eating at restaurants belonging to the same fast-food restaurant chain in Oregon and Michigan. . . . This report describes a clinically distinctive gastrointestinal illness associated with *E. coli* O157:H7, apparently transmitted by undercooked meat."

By this time, Tarr was a pediatrician and gastroenterologist at Children's, and he worked in a microbiology lab, where he shared an office with Dr. Peggy Neal, an internist doing clinical work on adults with bloody diarrhea. Neal had come from the CDC and was already doing cutting-edge research on *E. coli* that stemmed from taking stool cultures from adults with HUS. She had figured out how to test a stool sample for the presence of *E. coli* O157:H7. At the time, no states required hospitals or doctors to test for *E. coli* when collecting stool cultures from patients with intestinal sicknesses.

Taking a cue from Neal, Tarr arranged for all children admitted to Children's Hospital in Seattle with HUS to get their stools cultured for *E. coli.* That led to a series of studies by Tarr and his colleagues clearly linking *E. coli* to HUS and producing a statistic that about one out of every eight children that got *E. coli* O157:H7 ended up with HUS. Tarr emerged as a leading authority on the disease. But most public-health officials and physicians still knew little or nothing about it. That was what had Tarr worried. If children had already surfaced with HUS, statistically that meant there were probably close to fifty other kids out there with *E. coli* poisoning.

Suddenly the young intern appeared back in the doorway, panting.

"Where have you been?" Tarr asked.

"We've got three more kids with bloody diarrhea," he said, trying to catch his breath.

"Where did you go?" Tarr asked.

"Well, I went down to the emergency room."

Tarr was all ears.

The resident explained that he had leafed through the ER log for the past twenty-four hours. He discovered three kids that had come in with acute bloody diarrhea.

A chill raced down Tarr's spine. "We could be sitting on a disaster," he said.

The resident took a seat and Tarr picked up the telephone and called the state health department.

John Kobayashi had become the Washington State epidemiologist in 1982. A Japanese American with a biology degree from Rice, an MD from Stanford and a master's in public health from Harvard, the forty-four-year-old ran Washington State's public-health laboratory. Everything from drinking water to air quality in public buildings to infectious diseases fell under his area of responsibility. When his secretary told him that he had a call from Phil Tarr at Children's, Kobayashi told her to put it through. He had worked closely with Tarr on a variety of health scares. But *E. coli* was the thing that had really brought them together.

Shortly after Kobayashi took over the top public-health spot in Washington, the state had a small *E. coli* outbreak in Walla Walla, caused by bad ground beef served at a nursing home. Familiar with the outbreaks in Oregon and Michigan, Kobayashi convinced Group Health—the largest HMO in Seattle—to cooperate with the state in a study that involved testing for *E. coli* O157:H7 in all stool cultures taken by the HMO. A surprising discovery was made: it wasn't rare for people in the Seattle region to have *E. coli* O157:H7 in their intestinal tract when they had diarrhea.

As a result, Kobayashi pushed for two critical changes to the state's public-health laws, and Washington became the first state to make it mandatory for public-health officials and physicians to report cases of *E. coli* O157:H7 to the state health department. Then Kobayashi led the effort to raise the minimum internal cooking temperature in beef to 155 degrees in all restaurants licensed in the state. This represented a fifteen-degree increase over the federal government's recommended minimum temperature. Scientific studies had shown that *E. coli* could survive at 140 degrees, but not at 155 degrees.

Now, the minute Kobayashi heard Tarr's voice he knew there was trouble. "Something bad is happening," Tarr began, not bothering to say hello.

"What's going on?" Kobayashi asked.

"Here's some data for you, John," Tarr said, launching into a breakdown on the nine cases he knew about through the hospital.

To Kobayashi, what Tarr was describing had all the earmarks of a massive *E. coli* outbreak. Nine reported cases in less than twenty-four hours meant they were probably looking at the tip of a very large iceberg.

"I've never seen anything like this before," Tarr said.

That was what scared Kobayashi. If Tarr hadn't seen it, Kobayashi was pretty certain no one had. "This is terrible," Kobayashi said.

At this point, there was still no microbiological confirmation. But Tarr said he expected the results of the children's stool cultures back in less than twenty-four hours. He promised to call Kobayashi back the minute he had them in hand.

Later That Day

It was evening by the time forty-four-year-old Suzanne Kiner pulled into the parking lot at Woodinville Pediatrics, twenty miles from Seattle. Her nine-year-old daughter, Brianne, felt too weak to walk. Topping 250 pounds and with glasses and short wavy hair, Suzanne lifted her sixty-five-pound daughter from the backseat and carried her inside. Brianne had missed the previous day of school with a low-grade fever and stomach ache. Besides liquids, all Suzanne could get in her was raspberry popsicles. Then the diarrhea had started, along with the cramps that reduced Brianne to tears.

As soon as they got inside the clinic, Suzanne hustled Brianne to the bathroom. Once she got her situated on the toilet, Suzanne slipped a cup under Brianne's bottom to collect a urine sample. When she pulled the cup from underneath her daughter, the urine was blood red. So was Suzanne's hand.

"What is that, Mommy?"

"It's the raspberry popsicle you had earlier today," Suzanne said, trying not to panic.

Behind the thick lenses on her glasses, Brianne's eyes were full of fear.

Quickly patting her daughter dry and wiping her own arm with antiseptic, Suzanne stepped into the hallway with the cup of bloody urine in her hand. She held it above her head when she spotted the pediatrician. His eyes widened and he hustled toward her.

4

PROOF POSITIVE

The Next Day
Wednesday, January 13, 1993

PHIL TARR'S HUNCH WAS RIGHT. THE STOOL CULTURES FROM THE patients with bloody diarrhea came back positive for *E. coli* O157:H7. Now there was no doubt an outbreak was under way. The big question now was: How were all these kids coming into contact with *E. coli?* He called Kobayashi back, and the two men began brainstorming.

In the early stages of a bacterial outbreak, an epidemiologist's task is a lot like assembling a giant jigsaw puzzle. There are all sorts of disparate clues that have to be identified and connected. The longer it takes, the greater the number of people who fall ill. But unlike most food pathogens, *E. coli* can be lethal. "Time is not on our side with this disease," Tarr said.

Most of the previously documented *E. coli* outbreaks in the U.S. had been caused by ground beef. So Tarr and Kobayashi started with the assumption that beef was the vector. The fact that all nine victims lived far apart from each other ruled out the possibility that they'd eaten at the same place. That suggested a common retail source with wide distribution. The obvious candidates were chain grocery stores and chain restaurants. Step one toward identifying the right one would involve interviewing the parents of the sick children to find out where and what they'd eaten in the past week.

Meantime, Tarr said he had already notified the hospital's microbiology lab to make sure it maintained a deep supply of sorbitol MacConkey agar, which is used to test for *E. coli* in stool cultures. And he planned to convene a meeting with key hospital staff to brief them on the situation. The bigger problem was how to get word to all the pediatricians throughout the greater Seattle area to tell them what to look for. Very few of them had ever dealt with *E. coli* and didn't know how to spot its symptoms.

Kobayashi took on that task. He said he'd put together an urgent bulletin and have his office fax it to all emergency rooms throughout the Seattle area and beyond, notifying health officials to be on the lookout for symptoms and instructing them to notify the state lab at once if patients surfaced with bloody diarrhea.

After hanging up with Kobayashi, Tarr gathered his staff and gave them a quick primer on what they were dealing with. He gave the staff some tips:

1. From the time a person ingests *E. coli*, there's a two- to three-day incubation period.

2. During that time the toxin is proliferating and slowly being absorbed in the small bowel.

3. No antibiotics. Some emerging data suggested that patients with *E. coli* had worse outcomes if treated with antibiotics.

———

By the time paramedics removed Brianne Kiner from the ambulance and wheeled her into the ER at Children's Hospital, Suzanne Kiner was doing all she could to hold herself together. Brianne was writhing in pain, and the diarrhea just kept coming. So did the blood.

The ER was packed, chaotic, and loud. Suzanne's forty-five-year-old husband, Rex, a quiet, unassuming electrical engineer, began filling out paperwork. Suzanne stayed with Brianne as she was wheeled into a private room and her vital signs were taken. Her blood pressure was way up: dehydration had set in. Repeated attempts to get an IV line into a vein in Brianne's arm failed. The more the medic poked, the more Brianne shrieked in pain. Finally a senior nurse got the line in. More doctors and nurses kept coming into the room. And more and more wires and cords were running between Brianne and nearby monitoring devices.

Eventually, an epidemiologist wearing a medical overcoat and carrying a clipboard approached Suzanne with some questions, starting with where and what Brianne had eaten lately.

Hardly anything, Suzanne explained. Brianne had basically been on a liquid diet for the past four days.

Before that?

Before that was hard for Suzanne to remember. Her daughter was screaming in agony, making it hard to focus on what had been cooked for dinner five days earlier. The epidemiologist said she was less interested in what Suzanne had cooked than in whether Brianne had eaten at any restaurants lately.

Washington State epidemiologist John Kobayashi declared an E. coli *outbreak and notified Jack in the Box that it was the likely source.*

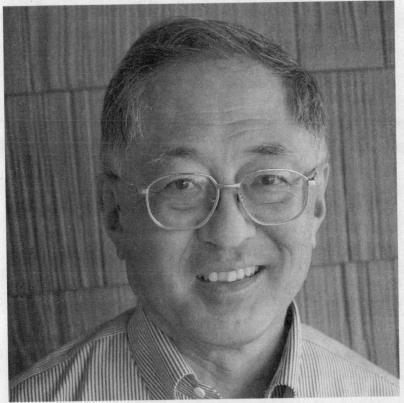

Photo by Morgan Robinson

That was an easier question. Jack in the Box, Suzanne told her. The epidemiologist asked if she was sure about that.

Suzanne was sure. They hardly ever ate out. But twice in the past week and a half Brianne had eaten out. And both times Jack in the Box was the place.

The epidemiologist asked if Suzanne knew what Brianne had eaten.

That was easy, too: a kid-size burger, french fries, and a milk shake. Same meal both times.

The epidemiologist noted all of this on a form and asked, "Are you sure Brianne didn't eat hamburgers anywhere else, such as McDonald's or Wendy's?"

Suzanne was sure.

By this point, Rex had entered the room and he noticed how the epidemiologist's eyes lit up when Suzanne mentioned hamburgers at Jack in the Box. Guilt swept over him. Rex had been raised on a beef cattle farm in Almira, Washington, where he'd seen cows get sick with diarrhea and then pass the illness on to the calves through the feeding process. Sometimes the calves died as a result. It was why his father had always stressed the motto "One hamburger, one cow," shorthand for slaughtering and processing one cow at a time." Rex rarely ate a hamburger after moving away from his father's farm, due to risks associated with large industrial meat-processing facilities. Yet he had let Brianne do it.

Friday, January 15, 1993

It had been less than three days since Kobayashi and Tarr determined they were dealing with an outbreak, and the number of confirmed cases was already up to thirty-seven, all of them children. Three children were in the ICU. Bed space and kidney-dialysis machines would soon be in short supply. It was imperative to find the source of the outbreak.

Kobayashi had narrowed his focus to a small handful of fast-food hamburger chains. Based on interviews with parents, all thirty-seven sick children had eaten at one in the past week. The problem was that they hadn't all reported eating at the same chain. Most of them—twenty-seven—had eaten at a Jack in the Box. But ten had reported eating elsewhere. Then there were some who had eaten at multiple fast-food chains, including Jack in the Box.

Jack in the Box, which had sixty-six restaurants throughout the state, was emerging as the most likely source, but Kobayashi couldn't publicly identify them without more evidence. He decided to notify Jack in the Box officials that the company was under suspicion and state health officials planned to inspect its restaurants throughout the Seattle area over the weekend.

Saturday, January 16, 1993

Suzanne Kiner was afraid to leave Brianne's side. It looked and sounded like her little girl was dying. Her breathing was rapid. She had deep pain in her chest. Her urine output had practically disappeared. Even her mental condition was deteriorating, and she was slurring her words when she tried to speak.

When the hospital transferred Brianne to the ICU for round-the-clock observation, Suzanne wanted answers. The doctors informed her that Brianne's stool culture had come back and definitely showed the presence of *E. coli* O157:H7. And her symptoms suggested she had hemolytic-uremic syndrome.

It was all foreign to Suzanne.

Basically, one of the doctors explained, Brianne's red blood cells weren't carrying enough oxygen to her vital organs, such as the kidneys, the liver, and the pancreas, not to mention the heart and the brain, which raised another set of concerns. On top of all this, Brianne's lungs were filling up with fluid, and a tube had to be inserted to drain them.

Suzanne didn't know what to say. Brianne was going downhill so fast. It seemed like no matter what the doctors tried, things just kept getting worse. She could only pray that the increased care in the ICU would make a difference.

But shortly after arriving in the ICU, Brianne suffered a seizure and stopped breathing. Doctors scrambled to resuscitate her. They gave her Dilantin intravenously, along with phenobarbital. Tubes were inserted in her chest. By the time doctors emerged to give Suzanne an update, Brianne was in a coma.

Suzanne had trouble swallowing. She wanted to scream, but all she could do was cry.

The doctors tried to keep her calm. The coma, one of the doctors explained, was actually a good thing, under the circumstances. Brianne had suffered a series of seizures that were putting tremendous strain on her little heart. The drugs were intended to stop the seizures and allow her heart to stabilize. Other drugs were being administered to combat her low blood pressure. And a mechanical device was helping her breathe.

All that was left to do now was watch and wait.

After the doctors left the room, Suzanne posted a handwritten sign above Brianne's bed: EXPECT A MIRACLE.

5

WE'VE GOT AN ISSUE

Sunday, January 17, 1993
San Diego, California

FIFTY-ONE-YEAR-OLD BOB NUGENT HAD REASON TO SMILE. AS PRESIDENT and chief operating officer of Jack in the Box, he had just led the nation's fifth largest hamburger chain through a year of extraordinary growth. In 1992 the company had opened sixty-three new restaurants, bringing the total throughout the country to 1,155. Seventy more were planned to open in 1993. One of the things driving sales was the chain's successful introduction of new items to its menu. The latest was the Monster Burger. Its promotion slogan was "So good it's scary."

With the company's stock doing well, Nugent's earnings were up, too. He and his wife had made a multimillion-dollar investment in a large piece of property in Rancho Santa Fe, the most exclusive suburb in the San Diego area. They planned to build their dream home there. The architectural design was finally complete, and the foundation was set to be poured within weeks.

Nugent was working his way through the Sunday paper in the living room of his condo when the phone rang. His wife told him it was Mohammed " Mo" Iqbal, the company's forty-three-year-old vice president of marketing. Nugent wondered why Iqbal was calling on a Sunday.

"We've got a problem up in Seattle," Iqbal said.

"What kind of problem?"

Iqbal wasn't entirely sure. The details were sketchy, but a bunch of kids had shown up at area hospitals with food poisoning, and the head of Washington's Department of Health had summoned Jack in the Box officials in Seattle to his office for an urgent meeting later in the day.

Nugent didn't like the sound of that.

Iqbal assured him that he had his hands around the problem. He had called his own meeting at corporate headquarters, in San Diego, for a few of the VPs in charge of quality control, operations, public affairs, and marketing. It was due to start in an hour. He didn't ask Nugent to attend.

"I'll be there," Nugent said.

He hung up the phone and turned to his wife. They had been planning to spend the day together. "I'm sorry," he told her. "I've got to go to the office."

"What's up?" she asked.

"There appears to be a problem with food poisoning up in Seattle. I don't think I'll be long."

His shirt collar open and his black hair slicked back, Nugent took his place at the head of a large conference table. He was flanked on both sides by VPs. Restaurant officials in Seattle were patched in via conference phone. Iqbal brought everyone up to speed on the latest information coming out of Seattle.

- At least three dozen kids were hospitalized with some kind of foodborne illness that was causing bloody diarrhea. A couple of kids were in intensive care.

- The state epidemiologist seemed convinced that contaminated hamburgers were the source of the illness.

- Interviews with the parents of the sick children had revealed that a lot of them had eaten at a Jack in the Box. But some of them had also reported eating at other fast-food chains in the Seattle area.

- Jack in the Box's regional managers in Seattle were scheduled to meet with public health officials early in the afternoon.

None of this made sense to Nugent, especially the part about kids being hospitalized and ending up in the ICU. For starters, food poisoning was a pretty common thing. Everyone got it now and again. It was a stomach bug that entailed the runs and, at worst, some vomiting. But after twenty-four to forty-eight hours it passed. "So why are kids in the hospital?" he asked.

Others wondered the same thing. No one had a good answer; except that the health officials were saying they were dealing with a pretty powerful bacterium.

"Well, what the *hell* is it?" Nugent wondered.

Again, no one could really say. But everyone was thinking the same thing: *should we stop the sale of our hamburgers in Seattle?*

Nugent felt that was way too premature. There were too many unanswered questions to lay all these illnesses at the door of one restaurant chain. There simply wasn't enough evidence to link the

---

Jack in the Box CEO Robert Nugent was blindsided by the news that his restaurant chain had served E. coli–*contaminated meat.*

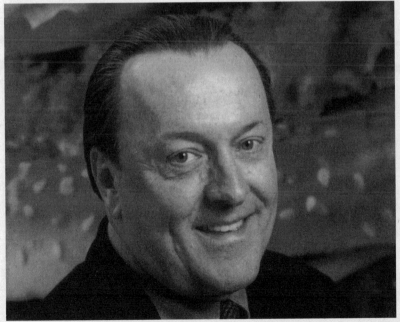

Courtesy of Jack in the Box Inc.

cause to Jack in the Box. At a minimum, Nugent wanted to wait for a report on the outcome of the meeting between the company's regional representatives and the state's health officials later in the day. Until then, he and everyone else at headquarters weren't going anywhere.

He stepped into his office and telephoned his wife at home. "I'm going to be here a while," he told her. "This is serious."

Later That Day
State Health Department
Seattle, Washington

"This does not look good," John Kobayashi told two Jack in the Box officials as a team of the state's top epidemiologists and microbiologists looked on at the state's public health laboratory.

Just the fact that they were meeting in a lab that tracked infectious diseases and pathogens had the Jack in the Box officials on edge. It was not where a food company would want to be. Kobayashi informed them that the state had positively identified thirteen different Jack in the Box restaurants where the sick children had eaten. As a result, he had a few questions.

"Where do you get your hamburger?" he asked.

"Well, we have sixty-six restaurants in this region," one of them said. "And all the hamburger comes from a warehouse in Tukwila."

Right away, something wasn't adding up. If all sixty-six restaurants got their meat from the same warehouse, why had only thirteen restaurants been implicated? Presumably, all sixty-six restaurants would have bad meat. In the back of his mind, Kobayashi couldn't help wondering if his team should be looking at something besides the beef.

He asked the Jack in the Box officials about their lettuce and bread. That went nowhere. Then he asked them about their employees, the people who handle the food. Another dead end. He even asked them about their supply trucks and delivery routes. Nothing suspicious there either. There appeared to be no smoking gun to explain why Jack in the Box's meat might be the source of the outbreak.

"How do you cook your hamburgers?" Kobayashi finally asked.

One of the restaurant officials explained the process. The patties are stored frozen in restaurant lockers. When a customer orders a burger, a patty is removed from the freezer and placed on the grill, at which point a timer is set. At the one-minute mark, the timer goes off, and a cook flips the burger and hits the one-minute timer again. "We've done our own internal testing in the food lab and the two-minute cook time meets the quality-assurance requirements," the official said. "All the burgers are being cooked to an internal temperature of 140 degrees."

"WHAT!" Kobayashi shouted, coming up out of his chair.

The Jack in the Box officials didn't see the cause for alarm.

Kobayashi repeated his question about internal temperature specifications for cooking beef patties.

Again, the official said 140 degrees, as required by the federal government's standards.

A number of the Washington health officials lowered their heads and covered their eyes. Kobayashi informed the Jack in the Box officials that one year earlier—on March 11, 1992—the Washington State Board of Health had adopted a new food service regulation: WAC246-215. It raised the minimum internal cooking temperature for ground beef to 155 degrees.

The restaurant officials insisted they knew nothing about the new standard.

Kobayashi assured them the company had been notified of this critical change a year earlier. And as a licensed operator within the state of Washington, the company had a legal duty to be in compliance with health standards.

The officials apologized profusely.

Kobayashi hit the table. "Look, we haven't proven that it's the hamburgers. But if you don't do something right now to fix this problem, we'll go public with it."

"We'll fix it," one of the officials said, explaining the company had an electronic communication network. "We can get this out to all of our outlets now and tell them to cook it longer."

Before the meeting broke up, Kobayashi directed a team of inspectors to lock down the Jack in the Box beef distribution center in Tukwila and remove packages of frozen beef for testing purposes. No meat was to leave the facility until the test results were in.

Second, he instructed his staff to prepare a public-health announcement to go out that evening, confirming an *E. coli* outbreak in the greater Seattle area. The announcement should admonish all consumers and restaurants to follow the state's guidelines and cook meat to an internal temperature of 155 degrees. But he agreed to leave Jack in the Box's name out of the announcement . . . for now.

"Damn it!" Bob Nugent shouted as he slammed his fist on the table. He'd just been briefed on what had transpired in the meeting in Kobayashi's office. Word that the company had not been in compliance with Washington's cooking-temperature regulation floored him. This was the first that Nugent had heard of a 155-degree requirement. That was what infuriated him. He was caught flat-footed. Seething, he turned to his vice president of quality assurance for answers on what the hell was going on.

Forty-two-year-old Ken Dunkley panicked the moment he learned what was up. Nine months earlier, the slender food scientist had been promoted from his position as director of research and development to the role of VP with responsibility for overseeing the quality of all food products sold at Jack in the Box restaurants. It was a promotion he took quite seriously. With a background in microbiology and a degree in food science from UC Davis, Dunkley had spent his entire career in the food industry. In his new managerial role, the safety of Jack in the Box's food fell within his purview. It scared him to death to discover that Washington had a 155-degree cooking regulation that was specifically intended to kill *E. coli.* That was the sort of thing he should have known about. But he hadn't.

With everyone at corporate headquarters scrambling to get a handle on what was happening, Dunkley retreated to his office and began tearing through files in search of any paperwork or official notices on the regulation. But he quickly reported back to Nugent that he and his staff were coming up empty. "We were really grasping for info about the Washington State action," Dunkley explained. "We were drawing blanks in terms of any citations on proper cooking."

The puzzling thing was that the FDA used 140 degrees as the temperature for killing *E. coli* in hamburger patties. Federal authorities were on record as saying that higher temperatures might result in overcooking. At this stage, all Dunkley could say for sure was that Jack in the Box was in compliance with the national standard.

Nugent was pissed. The state health department in Washington was on the verge of publicly linking Jack in the Box to a foodborne illness outbreak. They seemed to be pinning their conclusion on the fact that Jack in the Box's cooking procedure was in violation of state law. That was the bottom line coming out of the debriefing that followed the meeting with Kobayashi. But despite the cooking-temperature fiasco, Nugent couldn't accept the possibility that his company's meat was the problem. "It just *can't* be us," he said.

No one else in the board room wanted to admit it either. Jack in the Box was the oldest hamburger chain in the U.S. It had gotten its start in San Diego in 1950 just months before McDonald's was founded in San Bernardino. In all that time Jack in the Box had never been responsible for a foodborne illness outbreak. Its stellar reputation had been built on decades of consistent performance. All that would go up in smoke if it got linked to sick children in Seattle.

Dunkley was the one guy in the room who was convinced that Jack in the Box probably was the culprit. He took a clinical approach to the data coming out of Seattle: there were simply too many sick patients reporting that they had eaten at a Jack in the Box restaurant. From a scientific standpoint, that's no coincidence. He just wondered if the food source were something uncooked, like produce or a dairy product. The notion that there was a big enough presence of *E. coli* in the cooked beef to poison that many people had him scratching his head. His understanding of the organism was that it took a very high dose of live cells to poison a person. Even then, he thought, the worst case result was some temporary diarrhea. But clearly that wasn't the case in Seattle. That was what scared him. The company would be looking to him for expertise on *E. coli*, and he didn't have the answers.

Nugent had to deal with a more immediate question: should he recall all ground beef patties from the sixty-six restaurants in Washington State? If he didn't and the meat was, in fact, contaminated, he'd be putting more children at risk. On the other hand, if he issued the recall prematurely and the health department subsequently identified a different source, he would have effectively hung a Do Not Eat Here sign on all sixty-six stores and thrown into question the employment of more than two thousand Jack in the Box employees in that state.

Before taking such a step, Nugent wanted a definitive statement from Kobayashi that Jack in the Box was, in fact, the source of the outbreak.

But Kobayashi was still waiting on more lab results and was reluctant to make such a statement without solid evidence. A health official gets only one chance to be wrong when pinning an outbreak on a food company. After that, he's out of a job and possibly facing litigation.

With the state unable to pull the trigger, Nugent opted not to issue the recall. "I have to consider all the employees up there," he explained. "We start closing restaurants and I can't continue to pay employees without revenue coming in. They have those jobs because they need them. So if it isn't Jack in the Box and I prematurely make that decision, then shame on me."

Meanwhile, Nugent wasn't content to sit back and wait for information to come to him. He told Dunkley to go home and pack his bags, because Nugent wanted him on the next flight to Seattle. His assignment was to try to get to the bottom of what the hell was going on up there.

It was late Sunday night by the time Kobayashi checked in with Tarr for a status update from the hospital. The state had already issued a news bulletin indicating an *E. coli* outbreak. Tarr had talked to the press, too. But no source had been mentioned in the release and the media was clamoring for a name.

Meantime, the number of confirmed cases was up to forty-five. Word that Jack in the Box hadn't been cooking its meat to 155 degrees only solidified Tarr's convictions that beef was the vector. And with the number of cases continuing to mount by the day, Kobayashi knew he couldn't hold off any longer. He determined he'd call Jack in the Box's corporate headquarters first thing in the morning and notify them that he'd be issuing an updated media release formally tagging them as the source of the outbreak.

6

WHERE DID YOUR CHILD EAT?

Monday, January 18, 1993
Seattle, Washington

BOARDING THE EARLY MORNING FERRY, BILL MARLER FLIPPED A QUARTER to the guy selling newspapers, found a comfortable seat on board, and started scanning the headlines. "Bacterial sickness hits dozens of children," declared one. Intrigued, he read further.

> At least 45 people in Western Washington, most of them children, have fallen ill from an outbreak of a bacterial illness commonly linked to undercooked beef, the state Department of Health officials said yesterday.

Undercooked beef? Huh.

> The illness can cause severe complications, including kidney problems and excessive bleeding, the Health Department said in a news release.

Excessive bleeding from eating beef? Sounds bizarre.

> Several children became seriously ill and required hospitalization after being infected with the bacterium *E. coli* O157:H7. Four children ages eight months to nine years were in serious condition last night in the intensive care unit at Children's Hospital and Medical Center in Seattle. "It can be very serious," said Dr. Phillip Tarr of Children's Hospital. He said anyone with symptoms should get medical attention as soon as possible.

Bill noted the health department's recommendations for avoiding the bacterium: wash hands after using the toilet, changing diapers, or preparing food, and cook raw meat thoroughly before eating.

> The ground beef should be cooked to 155 degrees Fahrenheit. The
> specific cause of the illness has not been identified. The bacterium
> can be passed via person-to-person contact, although that probably
> isn't the primary mode of transmission in the latest outbreak, state
> epidemiologist John Kobayashi said.

Bill read between the lines. Even though the cause hadn't been identified, it sure looked and sounded like ground beef was the culprit. Why else tell people to cook it to 155 degrees? That was something Bill had never heard before. He wondered where all these kids had eaten that had made them sick.

That Same Morning
San Diego, California

Bob Nugent felt like hell when he arrived at his office Monday morning. Unable to stop second-guessing his decision to keep selling hamburgers, he'd hardly slept the previous night. Then he saw the morning headline out of Seattle. He had barely finished reading the story when he got a call from John Kobayashi. The lab had more conclusive data that clearly pointed the finger at Jack in the Box.

"We've done a case control study and we're confident in the results," Kobayashi told Nugent. "I'm going public with that information."

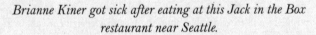

*Brianne Kiner got sick after eating at this Jack in the Box
restaurant near Seattle.*

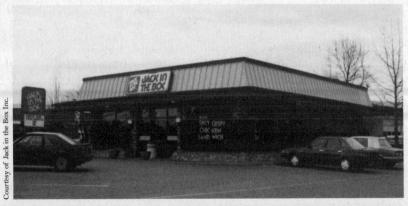

He also informed Nugent that the state was impounding the meat warehouse in Tukwila and seizing all twenty thousand pounds of beef stored there, a total of 250,000 frozen patties. The state no longer considered them fit for human consumption.

Nugent thought his company was getting screwed. He just wasn't convinced that the science was right. But he didn't argue. As soon as he hung up with Kobayashi he assembled a team of senior executives and issued two directives:

- Immediately suspend the sale of all hamburgers in all sixty-six Washington restaurants.

- Send the distribution people into all sixty-six restaurants and remove all unused frozen patties.

Ken Dunkley touched down in Seattle before 9:00 a.m. and went directly to the company's meat warehouse. There he met with state health inspectors who were on hand to lock the place down. After gathering more information on the state's cooking-temperature regulations, he met with some of the company's regional managers. Being in the Seattle area gave him a totally different feel for the scope of the crisis. Everyone he met with was talking about one thing—children who were deathly ill from an invisible organism. People were scared, especially the managers and operators of the local restaurants. Feeling desperate, Dunkley started racking his brain for someone the company could bring in to help them get a better handle on *E. coli*.

On the ferry ride home that evening, Bill bought the afternoon paper. It contained an update on the food poison outbreak. The state had tied it to Jack in the Box. And the restaurant chain had issued a recall on its beef.

When Bill walked through the kitchen door, Julie had the television tuned to the local news while she prepared dinner. The news anchor was talking about the food poison outbreak sweeping through Seattle.

"Jules, have you heard about this?" Bill said as he turned up the volume just in time to hear that Jack in the Box was closing stores and recalling twenty thousand pounds of meat.

"Wow," Julie said. "That's a lot of meat."

"Yeah, it's all over the newspaper."

Julie stopped what she was doing in the kitchen. The next report was about *E. coli.* She had never heard of it. Other than a brief mention in the paper, Bill hadn't either. The television reporter said that even scientists and doctors knew little about this new bacterium that apparently came from cows.

"That sounds really interesting," Bill said.

Julie thought *scary* was a better word.

Suzanne Kiner was slumped over a chair next to Brianne's bed, fighting back the urge to nod off. Any minute, she kept thinking, Brianne might open her eyes.

Her husband, Rex, had retreated to an ICU waiting room for parents. It was hard to find a seat in there. The place was filled with people whose children were suffering from HUS. But Rex was more overwhelmed by the scene in Brianne's room than this one. There were tubes and cords and wires running in and out of her body. His little girl was in a coma after eating a hamburger. It was just too much to process.

Suzanne had the opposite reaction. She avoided the waiting room for parents. She had tried lying down in there on the first night, but all she did was sweat on the horribly uncomfortable vinyl furniture. Meantime, parents had started calling that room the Death Room. Everyone in there had a child in critical condition. Suzanne got amped up just thinking about the place. Besides, there was no way she was leaving Brianne's bedside. Since arriving at the hospital three days earlier, Suzanne hadn't been home once to freshen up or change clothes. She was determined to go through her daughter's illness with her.

Suddenly a nurse entered the room and motioned for Suzanne to step out into the hallway. She had some news: Brianne was about to get a roommate—a little boy badly in need of kidney dialysis who had just been rushed to Children's from a hospital in Tacoma.

Diana Nole rode in the ambulance with her two-year-old son, Michael, from Mary Bridge Children's Hospital to Seattle. Although she was a unit secretary of an ER, Nole had never seen anything as horrific as her son's condition. Over a two-day span his diarrhea had gone from runny to all blood. The blood was so profuse that it went through his diapers and burned his skin. He became lethargic. His kidneys shut down. His abdomen swelled like a cantaloupe. And he couldn't urinate. Diana and her husband felt completely helpless. Doctors in Tacoma hoped the Pediatric ICU in Seattle could save him.

After a tear-filled, twenty-two-minute ride from one ER to another, Diana was whisked into a hospital room as doctors set Michael up in his bed.

It took a minute before Diana noticed the little girl in the next bed. She had tubes and lines in her body. Her eyes were recessed, her skin pale. "Hi," Diana said softly. "Looks like we get to share a room with you."

Before long, two-year-old Michael had tubes coming out of him everywhere—a catheter down below his groin to catch fluids, a chest tube to drain the fluid around his lungs, and a breathing tube. And he was being fed drugs through an IV to tamp down his dangerously high blood pressure.

Diana stayed beside him, kissing his cheek, stroking his golden hair, praying and wondering. *I'm his mommy. Why can't I fix this? Make everything better? Trade places with him?*

Already an emotional wreck, Suzanne cupped her mouth when she first spotted little Michael. His innocence brought tears to her eyes. *He looks like a little angel*, she thought to herself.

Then she looked at Brianne, unable to fight off a nagging thought, *Michael will live and Brianne will not*. Brianne just looked so much worse. It was hard not to compare.

But Michael was in critical condition, too. The *E. coli* had made a frontal attack on his intestines. Doctors feared that his underdeveloped immune system would succumb.

Once the doctors finally left the room, Suzanne met Michael's parents.

Young and blue-collar, the couple struggled to keep their emotions in check. "My name is Diana."

"I'm Suzanne Kiner."

"Where did your child eat?" Diana asked.

"Jack in the Box," Suzanne said.

Diana's lips came together tightly as she nodded her head up and down. Michael had eaten there, too.

Just like that, an instant bond had been formed between two mothers with dying children.

Diana revealed that Michael was her first.

Suzanne told her that Brianne was the youngest of three girls.

7

FLYING BLIND

Tuesday, January 19, 1993
Jack in the Box Headquarters

When under pressure, Bob Nugent tended to drop his head and close his eyes while squeezing the bridge of his nose between his middle finger and his thumb. The Seattle situation had him stressed out. The most frustrating thing was that he didn't know how to solve the problem. *E. coli* was a completely foreign term. He'd never heard of it. Ever. Yet health officials were telling him it was in his company's hamburgers and those hamburgers were making kids sicker than hell. At the same time, his corporate lawyers and PR people were giving him all kinds of advice on what to say—and mostly what not to say. But none of them knew a damn thing about *E. coli* either.

All Nugent knew was that in a matter of twenty-four hours he'd temporarily shut down sixty-six restaurants and recalled a hell of a lot of meat. Meantime, the number of sick kids kept climbing. It didn't take a degree in finance to realize that this equation added up to doom for a fast-food restaurant. The company had to find someone who could help explain this new bug and develop a plan for stopping it. He called Dunkley in Seattle for some direction.

By this time Dunkley had done some checking and come up with the name of an expert: Dr. David Theno.

The name meant nothing to Nugent.

Dunkley shared Theno's credentials—he was a PhD in food technology and food microbiology who had been doing research on *E. coli* for the National Cattlemen's Beef Association. He was also a member of the federal government's National Advisory Committee for Microbiological Criteria for Foods (NACMCF), a group impaneled by the USDA and the FDA to make recommendations on food safety. Before being asked to advise the federal regulators on food safety, Theno worked in the food-safety labs at Kellogg's and did a stint in the corporate headquarters for Armour.

"Get him down here," Nugent told Dunkley.

"You better get your ass back here."

Those aren't the words most guys want to hear when sitting

Jack in the Box hired food microbiologist Dave Theno to oversee the E. coli *crisis and to revamp the chain's food-safety protocols.*

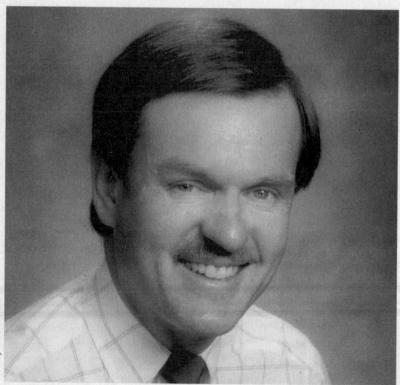

Courtesy of David Theno

poolside beside the wife, vacationing in Australia in January. But Dave Theno wasn't like most guys; he lived for calls like that. At 6'5" with broad shoulders and a thick crop of shiny blond hair, the founder of Theno & Associates (a consulting firm with the motto "If you are betting your business, you better get us"), was much more at home amongst cattle ranchers, wearing a cowboy hat and blue jeans over some well-worn, slip-on Timberland boat shoes, than at a resort. As soon as he got the message, he immediately called back to his office in Modesto, California. His colleagues told him they were hearing a lot of chatter about an *E. coli* outbreak in Seattle. They'd also checked with some of their well-placed sources in the food-safety and public-health communities and were told that the outbreak in Seattle might be linked to an emerging *E. coli* outbreak in San Diego.

"Oh . . . shit," Theno said. Nothing scared him more than the words *E. coli* and outbreak in the same sentence. He knew better than anyone in the food industry that *E. coli* was an emerging infectious disease in beef. There had been very few outbreaks. But the ones that had occurred had had very high morbidity and mortality rates. That's why the National Cattlemen's Beef Association had hired him to do microbial interventions in beef slaughter plants. They were trying to get ahead of the problem before consumers got scared away from beef. But it sounded to Theno like *E. coli* was no longer emerging— it had arrived. He cut his trip short and flew home immediately.

Theno had just landed his private plane and parked it in the hangar at the regional airport in Oakdale, California, when his phone rang. It was Ken Dunkley. Theno knew him, but not well.

"I don't know if you've heard," Dunkley said. "But there's an *E. coli* outbreak."

"Yeah, I've heard."

"Well, it's been tied to our restaurants, although we're not sure about that. The health department is still dancing around on some of that."

Theno asked him for the particulars.

While Dunkley spouted off what he knew, Theno jotted down notes:

- 45 cases of O157:H7.

- 27–37 cases tied to Jack in the Box.

- Washington epidemiologist: 206-361-2914.

- Cluster in San Diego.

- 2 cases in Oregon tied to Jack in the Box.

"Anyway," Dunkley said, "I know you know about lot about O157. Can you help us?"

"You probably need help yesterday, right?"

"Yeah."

They briefly discussed fees and Theno agreed to consult for $1,500 per day. If he was needed for more than a week, they'd draft a retainer.

"Well, we've got a lot of stuff to do here," said Dunkley, explaining that he was in Seattle and about to hop on a flight back to San Diego.

"All right," Theno said. "I can get down there tonight."

————————

The catheter attached to Brianne was intended to catch urine, but the liquid in the transparent bag looked more like red sludge. Meanwhile, the doctors were pumping more drugs into her: epinephrine and dopamine for low blood pressure and dobutamine to stimulate the heart. An echocardiogram revealed a build-up of fluid around the heart, and the left ventricle was not functioning properly. The doctors didn't like what they were seeing. Brianne was dying.

But Suzanne refused to see it. Not today. It was Suzanne's birthday. She was turning forty-five. "Brianne won't die on my birthday," she told the nurses. "She just won't do that. I know she won't."

The nurses admired her attitude, even if they doubted the prediction.

Amidst the bustle of medical staff, Suzanne leaned in close to Brianne, putting her lips to her daughter's ear. "This," she whispered, "is a six-inch brick wall and you are four-foot eight inches high. It's your choice. All you have to do is step over the brick wall."

Then Suzanne peeked at the monitors tracking Brianne's brain and heart activity. They hadn't changed. She looked back at Brianne, her eyes shut, her body still. *You can't die today. Not today. Not on Mommy's birthday.*

It was dark when Theno pulled up to the rear entrance of the Jack in the Box headquarters at 9330 Balboa Avenue in San Diego. Dunkley, looking haggard, met him there.

"What do you want to do first?" Theno asked.

"Well," he said, "I want to show you the data that we got from the health department."

They walked into a room where an array of faxes was spread out on a table in no particular order. Some were from the Washington State Department of Health. Others were from restaurant managers in Seattle who had received complaints from customers reporting illnesses. Theno thumbed through them.

"In the morning," Dunkley said, "you're going to be asked: 'Do you think this is us?' Because there's some people here that still aren't convinced."

"What else?" Theno asked, setting the faxes down.

"Then I'd like you to take a look at our beef specifications and tell me what you think."

Theno asked who their beef suppliers were.

Vons out of California and Portion-Trol out of Texas, Dunkley said.

"Where does the Vons meat go and where does the Texas meat go?" Theno asked.

Dunkley knew a lot about the Vons operation. The manager of the Vons plant had previously been in quality assurance at Jack in the Box. Dunkley showed Theno a map of the distribution routes. It was obvious that Dunkley was on top of the operation and how it worked.

He and Theno spent the rest of the evening tracing reported illnesses to meat suppliers. Then they reviewed all the faxes from the health department and the restaurants in Seattle.

It was clear that Jack in the Box hamburgers were contaminated with *E. coli.* The question was when and where did the contamination occur? It was way too early to reach conclusions about what was going on. But Theno had been around the beef industry longer than most and he had his suspicions about where to look. Health officials and the media were focused on Jack in the Box and its beef supplier, Vons. But Theno knew better. The problem undoubtedly started further up the food chain.

Virtually all conventional beef sold to consumers through restaurants and grocery stores comes from cattle that are raised on feedlots—huge industrial farms where hundreds of thousands of beef cows are confined to pens and deprived of their natural food source—grass. Instead, they are fed corn, a commodity made dirt cheap by government subsidies. Cows love the taste of corn, and it enables them to fatten up faster and produces the nice marbling in steaks.

But cows possess natural enzymes to break down grass, not corn. This subtle change in the diet of beef cattle has coincided with the growth of *E. coli* in the intestines of cows. This becomes a problem when beef cattle are butchered. If the intestine is accidently cut, *E. coli* can leak onto the carcass, a real possibility in slaughterhouses where upwards of six thousand cows are butchered per day. An even greater risk of *E. coli* contamination exists after slaughter when beef is ground into hamburger meat. The remains of hundreds of cows are ground through the same machines, ultimately ending up in large vats to be mixed all together. In this environment, *E. coli* can be widely dispersed, making it near impossible to trace back to one cow. All of this takes place before a company like Vons starts packaging and distributing to restaurants like Jack in the Box.

Privately, Theno had been warning federal regulators that *E. coli* posed a serious health risk to consumers. And he'd been telling the meat industry that the bug could one day threaten their business. But everyone from the USDA to the largest beef producers in the U.S. wanted to believe the occasional *E. coli* outbreak was a freak episode, the one-off problem rather than the symptom of a larger, industry-wide problem. It was just easier to blame the problem on human error, on poor handling procedures, careless hygiene, and improper cooking practices. But by the looks of the data coming out of Seattle, that theory no longer held water.

After a few hours of sleep, Theno returned to corporate headquarters early the next morning to meet the restaurant chain's top brass—Bob Nugent and Jack Goodall, the CEO of Foodmaker, Inc., the parent company to Jack in the Box. They met in Goodall's office.

"Do you think it is us?" Goodall asked.

"More likely than not, it is you," Theno said.

"What do you think we should do?" Goodall asked.

"Off the top of my head," Theno said, "the first thing you need to do is stop using Vons." The supply routes indicated that all the illnesses were in regions where the meat had come from Vons. "There are no illnesses coming in from the regions where the Texas meat has gone."

Terminating Vons as a supplier was an easy call for Goodall and Nugent. They asked what else they should do.

"Obviously I haven't looked at your cooking procedures yet," Theno said. "But you gotta make sure you are cooking to at least 155 degrees internally. But since I don't know how your grills are doing, I suggest you shoot for 160."

Both men nodded.

"Beyond that," Theno said, "Make sure all of the product is out of the field and sequestered."

Nugent piped in that the company had already issued a recall.

"But you need to go back and back again until you are absolutely positive there is *none* of that product in *any* store *anywhere*," Theno said. "That meat is like a time bomb out there."

Goodall still couldn't accept the idea that hamburger made kids so sick. "What else could be afoot here?" he asked.

Theno thought it was fruitless at this stage to look for another culprit besides beef. "In foodborne illness outbreaks you chase the rabbit you can see," Theno explained. "You should push down the investigatory lane that has the highest likelihood of being the source. It will quickly become apparent if you're going the wrong way."

But that didn't mean that Jack in the Box deserved all the blame. Theno briefly explained why he thought the contamination had taken place long before the hamburgers were delivered to Jack in the Box's warehouse.

Goodall thanked him for getting down to San Diego so fast and turned him over to Nugent, who led Theno next door to his office to discuss the scope of his role as a consultant. But as soon as they sat down it was clear Nugent didn't know where to begin. So much was happening so fast that he seemed disoriented.

"Look, I don't know much about you," Theno said. "But I know the meat industry, and I know this organism. And I know food-safety systems. I can help you."

"Just tell me how this could happen," Nugent said. "What's going on here?"

"Bob, I don't know today. But I know your meat specifications don't say anything about *E. coli*."

That's one of the things that scared Nugent. The company's internal protocols for transporting, storing, handling, and preparing ground beef included no mention of steps to take for preventing *E. coli* contamination.

"But you're like everyone else," Theno assured him. "No one is looking for it. Even the beef-industry guys don't know much about it."

That didn't make Nugent feel any better.

The one exception, Theno told him, was McDonald's, which had experienced two *E. coli* outbreaks in 1982.

Nugent had a blank look on his face.

Theno gave him the abridged version—in 1982, forty-seven people got *E. coli*, which was traced to McDonald's beef patties sold at restaurants in Michigan and in Oregon.

"Why in the hell haven't I heard about this?"

That was a good question.

The *New England Journal of Medicine* report didn't name McDonald's. But other publications, including the *New York Times*, had. Still, federal epidemiologists had treated the McDonald's cases as "isolated outbreaks" stemming from "an unusual type of dysentery." As a result, the public was in the dark about the danger associated with *E. coli* O157:H7 in meat. But insiders knew about it.

"What happened," Theno explained, "is that McDonald's did some fundamental research at the Food Research Institute up in Madison, Wisconsin." The principal researcher was a friend of Theno's, microbiologist Michael Doyle. "That's when McDonald's went to the clamshell grills and changed cooking procedures."

Doyle's research ended up being published in a number of obscure scientific journals. And shortly after that, Dr. Phil Tarr, up at Children's in Seattle, started his groundbreaking work on the effects *E. coli* has on children.

Listening to Theno, Nugent wondered why his VP Ken Dunkley had never told him any of this.

But that was a question for another day, because there were more immediate issues to tackle. For starters, at Theno's urging, Jack in the Box requested the microbial counts from the raw meat coming out of the plants that were supplying Vons. Meantime, Theno began looking for a new beef supplier to replace Vons. And that afternoon, Jack in the Box issued an emergency memo to all 1,155 restaurants with the words *ACTION REQUIRED* in bold letters across the top. The memo stressed the importance of fully cooking all hamburger patties and identified a series of steps to be implemented immediately. "Completing these steps is CRITICAL!" the memo read. "It is your responsibility to ensure that only fully cooked hamburger patties are served to guests."

Girl, 6, dies; undercooked meat blamed

By SUSAN DUERKSEN
Staff Writer

A 6-year-old San Diego girl has died and four other children have become seriously ill with a bacterial diarrhea linked to eating undercooked hamburger.

More cases may be going undetected, said San Diego County health officials, who are asking hospitals to check all patients with bloody diarrhea for the strain of E. coli bacterium that causes the severe condition.

The five confirmed cases were reported at Children's Hospital during the past three weeks. All the children ate hamburgers at a variety of fast-food restaurants within a few days before becoming ill, said Dr. Michele Ginsberg, county epidemiologist.

The health department is continuing to investigate the cause of the illnesses but has not planned extra inspections or restrictions on restaurants, said Dr. Donald Ramras, county public health officer.

"We need to know more before we harass people," Ramras said. "All I would say at this time is that thoroughly cooked meat is always safer, but I'm not going to stop going out to my favorite fast-food place."

Whether eating out or at home, he said, "It would be even more prudent now to eat your hamburger well-cooked."

Seattle is in the midst of a large outbreak of the same illness, with at least 66 confirmed cases in the past two weeks. Health officials in both cities said they have found no connection between the Seattle outbreak and the cluster of San Diego cases.

About 70 percent of the Seattle cases have been traced to eating at Jack In

See E. coli on Page B-11

E. coli

San Diego Union Tribune
Wednesday Jan. 20th 1993

Undercooked meat blamed in death

Continued from B-1

The Box restaurants, which obtained beef from a Von's store in the Los Angeles area, said Dr. John Kobayashi, Washington state epidemiologist. San Diego-based Foodmaker Inc. owns Jack In The Box.

The E. coli 0157:H7 bacterium is transmitted in contaminated food and water and, primarily, has been linked to undercooked beef. Any raw or rare meat can contain bacteria, but hamburger has more chance of becoming contaminated during the grinding process. Cooking kills the bacteria, which can also spread if individuals do not wash their hands after changing diapers or going to the bathroom.

Children's Hospital normally sees eight to 10 cases of E. coli diarrhea a year, and they usually occur in clusters, said hospital spokesman Mark Morelli. He and Ginsberg said they could not recall another death from the illness.

The 6-year-old girl died in late December of septic shock brought on by hemorrhagic colitis, which is caused by the E. coli strain, Morelli said. She had tested positive for infection with that bacterium.

Two other local children developed kidney problems; one was released from the hospital Tuesday after three weeks on dialysis and the other, a 2-year-old girl, remains on dialysis in serious condition.

The other two known cases were treated for the dehydration that is common with diarrhea.

An adult patient at Sharp Memorial Hospital in Kearny Mesa also had the condition in December, but no other hospitals have reported cases, Ginsberg said.

Unlike California, Washington state law requires doctors and hospitals to test for the E. coli strain and report cases to state health authorities. That policy has been in force since 1987, after two people died in an outbreak, Kobayashi said.

This press report marked the first time that Roni Austin heard that E. coli–*contaminated hamburger had caused the death of her daughter, Lauren.*

8

AN AWFUL SURPRISE

Wednesday, January 20, 1993
San Diego, California

RONI AUSTIN USED TO TELL PEOPLE SHE COULD DEAL WITH ANYTHING. But after Lauren had been gone for three weeks, Roni realized that that statement was no longer true. The grief was unbearable. It was hard to imagine how things could be any worse. Then she got a call from a neighbor.

"Have you seen the paper?" the neighbor asked.

"No."

"Well in the paper it says a six-year-old child died from uncooked beef."

Confused, Roni picked up the paper. "The six-year-old girl died in late December of septic shock brought on by hemorrhagic colitis, which is caused by the *E. coli* strain," the story reported. "She had tested positive for infection with that bacterium."

The article also reported that at least five other San Diego-area children were being treated at Children's Hospital for bloody diarrhea brought on by *E. coli*. But no official connection had been made to the ongoing outbreak in Seattle, which had reached a total of sixty-six confirmed cases. "About 70 percent of the Seattle cases have been traced to eating in Jack in the Box restaurants," the article reported.

With all that had been going on in her life, Roni had had no idea an outbreak was under way in Seattle. All she could think about now was Lauren. She put down the paper and picked up the phone to reach the reporter who wrote the article.

"This is Roni Austin," she began. "You wrote an article about my six-year-old that just passed away. I don't even know what *E. coli* is. What is it?"

By the time she got off the phone, Roni's grief was being overshadowed by anger. She was mad as hell at everybody: at the restaurant for selling bad meat, at the hospital for not telling her about the stool culture confirming the presence of *E. coli*, at the health department for failing to notify the public, and at the newspaper for running a story that felt like it violated the family's privacy.

Desperate, Roni called her attorney, Rick Waite. By this time, Waite had reached out to his friend Rob Trentacosta, one of the most respected trial attorneys in San Diego. Waite and Trentacosta had attended law school together. At Waite's urging, Trentacosta agreed to team up to represent Roni, although it was unclear what had caused Lauren's death. The story in the newspaper was starting to shed some light on that, however.

Then Roni provided one more piece of convincing evidence—a copy of the sales receipt from the night Roni's husband took Lauren out to eat for the last time. He'd been carrying it around in his wallet all this time. It was from Jack in the Box.

9

EXPIRED

Thursday, January 21, 1993
Children's Hospital
Seattle, Washington

IT WAS AFTERNOON WHEN TWO-YEAR-OLD MICHAEL NOLE WAS TAKEN to the operating room. After a series of EKGs had confirmed that he was losing cardiac functioning, doctors prescribed epinephrine to maintain his blood pressure. But no drug combination was working to slow down the expansion of his abdomen. It was dangerously enlarged and doctors hoped to reverse the problem with surgery.

Once surgeons opened up the toddler's abdomen, they discovered that all the tissue around the colon was dead. They had no choice but to remove his large intestine.

Suzanne Kiner was sitting with Brianne, praying that Michael would pull through. It was around midnight when Diana Nole entered the room. As soon as their eyes met, Suzanne knew the outlook was bleak.

During surgery, Michael had suffered two heart attacks. Both times doctors had been able to resuscitate him with CPR. But a neurological exam found no brain activity.

———————

When Diana and her husband were allowed in to see Michael, he had an incision from his neck to his groin. He opened his eyes once, just long enough for them to see the blue for the last time.

"You're Mommy's big boy," Diana said softly as she cried. "I will love you forever . . . and someday . . ."—she struggled to speak—"someday I will be with you forever in heaven."

It was early the next morning when Michael Nole's attending physician completed the Expiration Summary:

> After a prolonged discussion between Dr. Elliot Krane and the family, decision was made to maintain support and follow Michael's neurological examination as well as his response to inotropes. As inotropes were increased, the decision was made by the family and the Intensive Care Unit Team to withdraw support. Michael expired at 5:25 AM on the morning of 1/22/93.

Diana Nole left the hospital with Michael's blanket, his shoes, a choo-choo train, and a lock of his golden hair given to her by the attending nurse.

The Seattle media seized on the news that the outbreak had claimed the life of a child. By midday the national media had picked up the story. Before the end of the day Wall Street got hold of the bad news out of Seattle, too. Shares of Foodmaker, Inc.—Jack in the Box's parent company—started plunging. Before the closing bell at the New York Stock Exchange, the Securities and Exchange Commission indefinitely suspended trading in Foodmaker's stock. By the end of the day, a prominent member of Foodmaker's board was calling for Nugent to be fired. It was important, he argued, to send a message to Wall Street that executives would be held accountable for this mess.

Dave Theno was seated at his desk, talking on the telephone in his new office at Jack in the Box headquarters when he looked up and saw Nugent coming through the door. He had bags under his eyes and his mercurial temper had been overcome by melancholy. "I'll call you back," Theno said, hanging up the phone and looking up at Nugent.

"We have a child that's died," Nugent said.

Theno was already aware of Michael Nole's death. It was hard to know what to say.

"Who the hell thought we were dealing with a product that had the potential to kill children?" Nugent said. "Who the hell thought that! Never in my wildest dreams did I think that potential was there."

Before joining Jack in the Box, Nugent had worked for Ponderosa, a national chain of steak houses. "We had this Number Four dinner at Ponderosa," he explained. "It was a half-pound ground beef patty. People always ordered it rare. That's the industry I came from."

Theno could relate. His background was in the same industry.

"Then we had the 40-140 rule," Nugent continued. "You had to store meat below 40 and cook above 140. This precluded bacteria. But even if bacteria did develop, so you had upset stomach and diarrhea for a day or two. But people *dying*?"

Nugent shook his head and plopped down in a chair across from Theno. "I can't believe this has happened," he said.

Theno took a deep breath before trying to explain why *E. coli* is so much more serious than *Salmonella* and other well-known foodborne illnesses that have been around longer. "If 1,000 people get sick with *Salmonella* you might have one person die and that's because the person is elderly and has a compromised immune system," Theno explained. "You get 100 people sick with *E. coli* and 5 or 10 of them may die."

"Holy shit," Nugent whispered, turning his head from side to side in frustration. "How bad is this going to get?"

"Bob, I don't know how much of this bad meat has been consumed. But everyone who has consumed it has the potential to get this. So there could be five hundred illnesses, I don't know."

Nugent's face went pale. It sounded to him like *E. coli* might threaten the entire business model of selling fast-food hamburgers. "How can we sell hamburgers again? How can we even do this?"

"We can put together a comprehensive program that will work with your beef suppliers," Theno said.

"Will the program insure that this never happens again at a Jack in the Box restaurant?"

"Never is a big word. Look, Bob, this is science. You can't test raw materials 100 percent. But I can give you a program that is a hell of a lot better than what you've got now."

That's what Nugent wanted.

"But I gotta tell you," Theno warned, "if I do this for you, we're going to change manufacturing; we're going to change specifications; we're going to change restaurant processes. The whole world is going to look different."

"Show me what that world will look like."

Theno promised to try to have something put together within thirty days.

Michael Nole's death was still fresh on Suzanne Kiner's mind when doctors rushed Brianne into surgery to undergo the same procedure that Nole had failed to survive. Brianne's bowel was bleeding internally and the infection was spreading. The surgery team planned to remove her entire colon and divert the fecal stream from her rectum and anus to a colostomy bag. Since the colon was where the *E. coli* bacterium was producing the deadly toxin attacking Brianne's body, doctors hoped that by removing the colon they'd eliminate a great deal of the toxin from her system.

But during the procedure, complications arose. Brianne developed severe hypotension—the blood pressure to her heart and brain dropped way off. Powerful drugs were administered to improve her cardiac functioning. And a ventilator kept her breathing—barely. By the time it was over, Suzanne was a wreck. How much more could her little girl take?

Brianne Kiner had to undergo emergency surgery to remove her colon. During the procedure she developed severe hypotension.

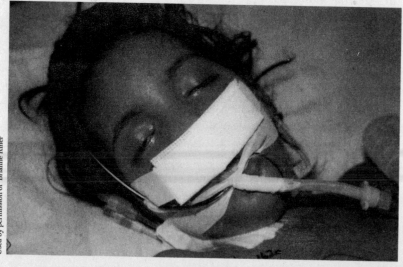

10

IT PAYS TO BE NICE

Tuesday, January 26, 1993

"THE JACK IN THE BOX POISONINGS." THE BANNER HEADLINE was impossible to miss, along with the series of stories under it. The outbreak had become the biggest story in the city. After reading a heartbreaking story about how nine-year-old Brianne Kiner remained in a coma, Bill Marler studied the full-page ad Jack in the Box had taken out. "This is a horrible event, and all of us at Jack in the Box extend our prayers for a complete and speedy recovery to everyone who has experienced this illness." The company pledged to establish a one-hundred-thousand-dollar foundation in memory of any child who died in the outbreak. The ad also reiterated all the corrective steps the restaurant chain had taken, such as replacing the hamburger supply, raising cooking temperatures, and retraining employees.

Someone not directly impacted by the outbreak might be impressed by the restaurant chain's pledge. A parent with a child on life support might curse the company for doing too little too late. But Bill couldn't help thinking three things: First, only big companies in big trouble took out full-page ads to apologize and give away money. Second, the ad implied that the company anticipated more children would die before all was said and done. Third, by advertising what it was doing correctly now, the company was essentially admitting what it was doing incorrectly before—using inadequately trained employees who were undercooking contaminated meat.

When he reached his office, Bill tucked the ad in a file. Then the receptionist notified him that a former client was on the line, a woman who had slipped and fallen a few months back while working at a car dealership and had wanted Bill to sue the dealership. Bill remembered her. He had talked her into forgoing a lawsuit in favor of pursuing workman's compensation. Bill had made nothing off the case. But the woman recovered her lost wages and had all her medical bills paid.

He wondered what she was calling about this time.

"Hi, Bill," the woman said. "Hey, listen, my friend's kid is sick with this *E. coli* thing."

Bill leaned forward in his chair, gripping the phone tightly and pressing it against his ear. "You mean from the Jack in the Box outbreak?" he asked.

The woman said yes and shared what little she knew—that the child had been hospitalized with really bad abdominal pain and that a doctor had said it was caused by bad meat. The parents were overwhelmed with medical and legal questions. "Is it okay if I have her call you?"

Later that morning Bill's phone rang again. The woman on the other end introduced herself as Karen Gragg, the friend of Bill's former client. After some small talk, Bill asked about her situation.

Gragg explained that on January 7 she had taken her daughter Lorissa to a Jack in the Box restaurant in Tacoma. Three days later Lorissa had become violently ill and was hospitalized at Mary Bridge Children's Hospital with food poisoning symptoms. A physician subsequently told Gragg that her daughter's illness was the result of an *E. coli* infection. And public-health officials had indicated that the source of the *E. coli* was contaminated hamburger meat. The family was hoping to at least recover medical expenses.

Bill asked a series of follow-up questions then promised to get right back to Gragg. He hung up, hardly able to believe he'd gotten a call like that. The *E. coli* outbreak dominated every newscast. Lawyers were falling over themselves to get in on the action against Jack in the Box. One attorney had gone as far as to take out an ad in the newspaper, inviting parents of sick children to hire him. The ad had made Bill cringe. Stunts like that were what gave personal-injury lawyers a reputation for ambulance chasing.

Yet Bill appeared poised to land a client by way of a personal referral. Eager to tell someone the news, he rushed down to the office of the firm's managing partner, Lynn Sarko. But Sarko's secretary said he was out. Then Bill spotted twenty-eight-year-old Mark Griffin, an associate. He maintained the office next to the managing partner's.

"Hey, Griff, guess what?" Bill said, bursting into Griffin's office and launching into a blow-by-blow account of his conversation with Gragg.

Chubby with a gregarious smile and neatly trimmed beard that handsomely hugged his face, Griffin immediately saw the possibilities. The Jack in the Box outbreak was the biggest story in town. The prospect of landing a client from the outbreak could mean big things for the firm.

Bill agreed.

But Griffin wasn't thinking about just one client. He was thinking about lots of clients. Griffin was part of the firm's complex-litigation unit and he worked almost exclusively on class-action lawsuits. Lately, most of his time had been dedicated to the *Exxon Valdez* oil spill. Keller Rohrback represented hundreds of commercial fishermen and canners who had been put out of work by the Exxon's oil spill. Jack in the Box's crisis presented a similar opportunity.

"This could be a great class-action case," Griffin said.

Bill had never worked on a class-action suit. He understood the concept—a single action brought by a group of individuals suffering similar injuries and seeking similar relief from the same wrongful conduct—but he only had one potential client.

But one client was all that was required to file a class-action suit. Other injured persons could subsequently be added to the complaint. The important thing was to file quickly, as other law firms were sure to pursue class-action suits, too. Ultimately, a judge would certify one class of plaintiffs and select one firm to represent them. Often, the first one to file was the firm that got chosen.

Bill agreed to call Gragg back right away and gauge her interest.

Griffin turned his attention to research. He wondered whether the courts had ever approved a class-action approach in a food poison outbreak. He reached for a copy of *Newberg on Class Actions*, a multivolume treatise that contained information on every major class-action case filed in the U.S. Flipping to the pocket part at the back of one of the volumes, he found two foodborne illness outbreaks that had become class-action complaints. Both had arisen from outbreaks aboard cruise ships. In each instance the class-action approach had made perfect sense—all the victims had gotten sick at the same time in the same place by eating the same food. And the illnesses had been relatively short-term and hadn't involved fatal injuries.

But the cruise ship cases weren't perfectly analogous to the *E. coli* outbreak. The biggest difference was the severity of the injuries. In the *E. coli* outbreak the injuries ranged widely, from mild diarrhea to death. But that didn't concern Griffin. He was just pleased to see that there was some precedent for what he had in mind.

Bill came back with good news, too. He'd reached Gragg and she seemed willing to be part of a class of victims. Before going any further, Griffin wanted to get approval from the firm's managing partner.

———

No one at Keller Rohrback had doubted the abilities of Lynn Lincoln Sarko when he joined the firm at age thirty in 1986. Tall with bushy hair and an intense gaze, he came from the U.S. attorney's office in Washington, DC, where he prosecuted big corporations in violation of antitrust and federal racketeering laws. Before that he clerked for the U.S. Court of Appeals in the Ninth Circuit. An experienced trial lawyer with an MBA in accounting and a mind that worked like a steel trap, Sarko started the complex-litigation unit at Keller Rohrback, dealing with antitrust and mass torts.

Within two years he got promoted to partner and filed his first class-action suit on behalf of nuclear-power plants and some conventional-fuel power plants that had been victims of a price-fixing conspiracy. Then, in 1989, Sarko got besieged with calls from lawyers representing individual fishermen who had been put out of business by the *Exxon Valdez* oil spill. Ultimately, Sarko ended up with over five hundred clients—fishermen, cannery operators, and owners of small maritime businesses—and filed a class-action suit against Exxon. The power-plant case and the Exxon case promised to be two of the biggest fee generators in Keller Rohrback's history. So in 1991, the firm made

Sarko its managing partner. He was just thirty-four, making him the youngest managing partner in the firm's long history.

Griffin worked alongside Sarko in the complex-litigation unit. They had become quite close and trusted each other instinctively. At all times they knew each other's whereabouts. Griffin punched in Sarko's cell phone number and reached him in Philadelphia, where he was working on the power-plants lawsuit. First Griffin reported that Marler had a prospective client from the *E. coli* outbreak, someone willing to serve as a class representative. Then he shared the result of preliminary research on the cruise-ship cases.

Sarko was not easily impressed. But he had a lot of respect for Griffin's ability to identify cases that were attractive for a class-action approach. And Sarko had never heard Griffin talk so fast or sound so giddy. Acknowledging a potential upside to a class-action approach against Jack in the Box, Sarko had a couple of initial thoughts on the idea: Consumer negligence cases involving child victims were very high-risk for law firms. More often than not, the injured families recovered very little money. That was because powerful insurance and business interests combined to punish the little guy. Whether it was lead in toys or defectively manufactured car seats, the playbook was the same: after a bunch of children suffered relatively minor injuries, the corporation responsible for the damage would pretend to help the injured consumers by having its insurance company pay out small sums in exchange for the consumers' signing a release that would protect the corporation from further liability. Then the companies would just ride out the public relations storm. These cases just didn't generate adequate legal fees.

Unfortunately, without competent legal representation, a consumer was wasting time by taking on a big corporation. And without an ability to extract a big-enough settlement, lawyers were wasting their time taking on the complaints of individual consumers. In Sarko's view, the class-action approach was the only way to overcome this problem. By grouping together a large pool of victims, a plaintiffs' lawyer could create leverage for his clients and secure ample legal fees for his time.

After a brief discussion, Sarko agreed with Griffin's approach. But as the firm's managing partner, Sarko had other things to consider. A class-action suit against Jack in the Box would ultimately end up in the laps of insurance companies, which would be required to shell out the money to settle the claims. That posed a problem. Keller Rohrback was still among the top insurance-defense firms in Seattle. No doubt some of their largest clients would push back against the idea of Keller Rohrback's seeking to extract large settlements from insurance companies.

Sarko figured he'd cross that bridge later. He gave Griffin and Marler the green light to go forward.

Bill agreed to set up an appointment to meet with the Gragg family the next day.

11

TELL ME ABOUT *E. COLI*

Thursday, January 28, 1993
Children's Hospital
Seattle, Washington

WHEN A JOURNALIST ASKED DR. PHIL TARR WHAT IMPACT THE LOSS OF a child had on the hospital's doctors and nurses, he put it this way—it's like trying to quantify infinity multiplied by one thousand.

At 8:30 a.m. on January 28 the outbreak claimed its second child at Seattle's Children's Hospital. Two-year-old Celina Shribbs had succumbed to heart failure. Tarr was pretty certain she wouldn't be the last child to die in the outbreak. The number of confirmed illnesses was up to 250. If the percentages held, at least 31 of them would get HUS. And a handful of those would not survive.

The situation was too grim to dwell on. Instead, Tarr tried dwelling on the positive. If the recall of Jack in the Box meat had been delayed even a couple more days, there would be many more illnesses and undoubtedly more deaths. The state health department's test results had revealed "massive amounts of contamination in raw hamburger" taken from the restaurant chain's distribution center in Seattle. Only about a third of that batch had reached the restaurants before the state announced the outbreak. That meant two-thirds of the meat had been caught in time.

That was slim consolation, but it spoke to the importance of Washington's mandate that health officials report cases of *E. coli* to the health department. Washington was one of only a handful of states that required such reporting. And the staff of Children's Hospital in Seattle had by far the most expertise in the country when it came to treating an outbreak. If this had happened anywhere else in the U.S., the damage could have been far more catastrophic.

That Same Day
Jack in the Box Headquarters

Shortly after Bob Nugent learned that a second child had died in Seattle, he got word from his PR people that the Associated Press had put out a story on its wire service under the headline "Food Poisoning Nightmare Spreads Across West." It reported that the outbreak was now in four states and "had produced symptoms ranging from bloody diarrhea and intense abdominal pain to stroke-like bleeding in the brain and irreversible damage to intestines and kidneys."

Nobody would feel like eating a hamburger after reading a story like that. But the worst part, at least from the perspective of Jack in the Box's lawyers, was something Nugent had told the AP reporter. "Nugent," the story reported, "has said the company was in violation of Washington state cooking regulations because it didn't know the state last May required that burgers be cooked to an internal temperature of 155 degrees, highest in the nation."

Jack in the Box had hired San Diego trial lawyer Fred Gordon to sue its meat supplier Vons. Under the Meat Inspection Act—a federal law that spells out the food codes—it is a breach of warranty to sell or distribute food that is contaminated or adulterated. Gordon intended to argue that Vons had violated the law by selling contaminated meat to Jack in the Box. But when Gordon read the statement the AP story attributed to Nugent, he wasn't happy. It sounded like an admission of negligence. Vons's lawyers could have a field day using Nugent's words to support the meat supplier's claim that if the restaurant had simply cooked the meat to the law's specifications, no one would have gotten sick.

Just thirty-six, Gordon was cocky beyond his years and had no hesitation telling a fifty-one-year-old corporate executive making seven figures to shut his mouth.

"Shit, this is going to hurt my case," he told Nugent.

"What the hell was I going to say? The fact is that we didn't know."

Gordon advised him not to talk about it again. Just leave it alone.

That advice was fine for future media interviews. But right after the AP story ran in newspapers nationwide, Jack in the Box's legal department received a subpoena from Congress. The U.S. Senate's subcommittee over agriculture and nutrition had scheduled a hearing titled "Food Safety and Government Regulation of Coliform Bacteria." The Senate wanted Nugent to testify.

Everyone at corporate headquarters knew what that meant. Jack in the Box's problems were no longer going to be confined to Seattle and a few western states. The whole country was about to learn about *E. coli* through a congressional hearing that focused on Jack in the Box. From a PR standpoint, nothing good could come of this. The lawyers felt the same way.

Nugent had one week to prepare. The hearing was set for February 5 in Washington.

Ken Dunkley was relieved to have Dave Theno around. Theno had assumed all the responsibility for dealing with the scientific questions about *E. coli*, leaving Dunkley to focus on a series of new procedures being implemented by the company, such as increased cooking temperatures for beef in every Jack in the Box restaurant in the country. At the same time, Dunkley was calling his counterparts at other national fast-food chains to see how they were dealing with *E. coli*. He discovered that everybody he talked to was just as baffled as he was. One guy said he just thanked his lucky stars that it wasn't his restaurant that had gotten hit with this. His point was that it could have happened to anybody.

Dunkley appreciated the support of his colleagues, but it did little to relieve his sense of guilt. He couldn't get over the idea that he should have known about the law in Washington. Normally a detail-oriented, studious type, he was disturbed by the thought that he might have missed something. That was essentially what he had said when asked by the company's in-house attorneys who were trying to figure out who had known what about the cooking-temperature regulation.

Dunkley's wife knew that he hadn't been sleeping and he'd been practically living at the office. One evening she suggested they take their daughters out for dinner. Their girls were ages four and seven and they preferred a fast-food hamburger place near their home. At the restaurant, the girls ordered children's meals with hamburgers. One of them bit into her hamburger and discovered it was pink in the middle. "Daddy, is this okay to eat?"

Dunkley examined it. In the past he would never have worried about some pinkness in a hamburger. All of a sudden, a simple question from his child had him stymied. *Should I let her eat it?* he thought.

His mind immediately drifted to all the children who were hospitalized in Seattle. They were there because they had eaten undercooked hamburgers. It became brutally clear to him just how easily the same thing could happen to his own daughters. He couldn't stop telling himself that this whole epidemic might have been avoided if he had just been more vigilant in his work.

———————

Mark Griffin couldn't help laughing as he and Bill pulled into the parking lot at the Poodle Dog Restaurant, a greasy spoon with an old, partially burnt-out neon sign in front. Only Bill would arrange to meet a client at a place like this. Bill knew the diner from his law school days in Tacoma at the University of Puget Sound.

Inside, Bill and Griffin squeezed into a booth opposite Karen Gragg. Bill made small talk before Griffin removed a document from his binder. It listed the duties of a representative of a class. As he would with a client signing documents at a mortgage closing, Griffin walked Gragg through each requirement: A plaintiff had to be willing and able to represent the class. That meant, Griffin said, the plaintiff would devote time and resources of her own for the good of the larger group. Next, the head of a class was required to hire lawyers who had experience litigating class-actions.

One by one, Griffin worked through the list and asked if Gragg had any questions. She turned her head from side to side. Then Griffin handed her a pen and showed her where to sign.

Next, Griffin went over the retainer agreement. Bill fidgeted. The business side of personal-injury law always made him uneasy. The bar association required lawyers working on a contingency-fee basis to have a signed agreement with the client. Bill couldn't help feeling uneasy that he was forming a relationship with the parents of a sick child and he was going to benefit financially as a result.

While Gragg looked over the agreement, Bill put it in simple terms. "If we don't get any money for you, then you don't owe us any money." Gragg signed the retainer and pushed it back across the table.

That afternoon, Griffin began drafting the civil complaint back at the office. Bill took a cab across town to the library at the University of Washington's medical school, where he bounded up the steps and approached a reference-desk librarian.

"Hi, I need information on *E. coli*," he said.

The librarian smiled. "You're working on the outbreak, aren't you?"

Grinning, he nodded.

"Well, there isn't much out there on the topic," she said. "But c'mon back."

She led him to the stacks and recommended a textbook on bacteriology. While the librarian went to retrieve some medical journal articles, Bill immediately started looking up definitions. He started with *E. coli*.

> A bacterium known as *Escherichia coli* that has hundreds of strains, some of which produce a powerful toxin that may cause severe illness. Most strains of *E. coli* are harmless and live in the intestines of healthy people and animals. *E. coli* is differentiated from other strains by specific markers found on its surface.

He glanced at the medical illustration next to the definition. It depicted tiny hair-like structures that attach to a person's intestinal lining. He continued reading.

> It is also referred to as diarrheagenic *Escherichia coli* or non-Shiga toxin-producing *E. coli* and was first identified as a cause of foodborne illness in the United States in 1982.

E. coli has been around since 1982? Up until a couple of weeks earlier Bill had never heard the term. He couldn't help wondering why the public knew so little about this. Then the librarian came back with some articles from medical journals. The one on top was from the *New England Journal of Medicine*. Bill scanned the abstract.

> We investigated two outbreaks of an unusual gastrointestinal illness . . . characterized by severe crampy abdominal pain, initially watery diarrhea followed by grossly bloody diarrhea, and little or no fever. It was associated with eating at restaurants belonging to the same fast-food restaurant chain. . . . This report describes a clinically distinctive gastrointestinal illness associated with *E. coli* O157:H7, apparently transmitted by undercooked meat.

Bill was intrigued. A fast-food restaurant chain served undercooked hamburgers leading to bloody diarrhea and a lot of sick people. It sounded just like the Jack in the Box situation, only ten years earlier. He had more questions:

- Which fast-food restaurant was involved in the 1982 outbreak?

- Why hadn't the public ever heard about this outbreak?

In the body of the article he noticed that the CDC had studied the stool specimens from the 1982 outbreak. And the U.S. Department of Agriculture Animal Laboratories had also been involved in studying the cause of the outbreak. It looked like the CDC and the USDA had known way back in 1982 that deadly *E. coli* could be transmitted through hamburger. It seemed to Bill that if one of the most popular foods in America had had a health risk associated with it, consumers should have been made aware of it.

He went back to the textbook definition of *E. coli* and looked up the causes and symptoms: diarrhea, bloody diarrhea, and hemolytic-uremic syndrome.

Hemolytic-uremic syndrome? He'd seen that term in the newspaper, but not well defined. He looked it up.

> Hemolytic-uremic syndrome, commonly known as HUS, is a potentially deadly disease that sets in after the bloody diarrhea and results in kidney failure.

Bill repeated the pronunciation. "HEE-mo-litic you-REE-mic syndrome." He figured he'd better be able to say it properly, because he planned to have a press conference as soon as his case got filed.

One of the journal articles furnished by the librarian came from the *Journal of Pediatrics* and was titled "Long-term outcome and prognostic indicators in the hemolytic-uremic syndrome." The lead author was Dr. Richard Siegler, a nephrologist in the division of infectious diseases at the University of Utah's School of Medicine. Over a ten-year period, Siegler had monitored sixty-one children treated for HUS at Primary Children's Medical Center in Utah. He found that children with HUS can suffer chronic disease that lingers for years and goes as far as causing the central nervous system to dysfunction. One line from the study jumped out at Bill: "Abnormalities sometimes appeared after an interval of apparent recovery. . . . Physicians should therefore be cautious in assuming recovery from HUS on the basis of a single evaluation."

This sounded worse than anything Bill had read in the press. He started scribbling down notes. Damages are a key element of any personal-injury claim, and a plaintiff's suit has to indicate what it would take in financial compensation to make the victim whole. That was going to be nearly impossible in cases where an *E. coli* infection led to HUS, since it appeared the medical ramifications to a child could extend for years. To explain all this to a jury, Bill was eventually going to need an expert. And from what he could see from the literature, Dr. Richard Siegler was the expert among experts when it came to HUS and long-term illness.

It wouldn't be long, Bill figured, before all the other lawyers getting involved in lawsuits against Jack in the Box would come across Siegler's name. Whoever got to Siegler first had the best chance of securing him as an expert witness.

Bill started popping coins in the Xerox machine. Then he tucked the copied journal articles in his bag and rushed back to his office to track down a phone number for Dr. Siegler in Utah.

When Dr. Richard Siegler first joined the faculty at the Utah School of Medicine, the Department of Pediatrics had no pediatric nephrology division. So Siegler started one. And over a ten-year period he helped turn University of Utah Hospital into the go-to place for children suffering kidney failure. He became an expert on *E. coli* because it started showing up in children as a major cause of kidney failure.

Bill knew none of this when he called Siegler's office in hopes of talking to him. He introduced himself to Siegler's secretary as a lawyer in Seattle working on the *E. coli* outbreak. She was familiar with the situation. Unfortunately, Dr. Siegler was out of the office.

Bill said it was urgent he speak to Siegler as soon as possible. The secretary suggested Bill speak to Dr. Andrew Pavia, the chief of the hospital's Division of Pediatric Infectious Diseases. Pavia had collaborated with Siegler on research into the effects of *E. coli* among children.

Pavia was in and took Bill's call. And he was well aware of the situation in Seattle. "I'm hoping you or Dr. Siegler can help me understand what's going on," Bill began.

Pavia agreed to help. He informed Bill that he and Siegler were nearly ready to publish a groundbreaking study on hemolytic-uremic syndrome that was based on their observations of children in Utah. In all they had looked at 157 cases where children had suffered HUS, going all the way back to the early 1970s.

The 1970s?

Yes, Pavia explained. The study was a twenty-year, population-based study.

But Bill had read in the *New England Journal of Medicine* that the first reported cases of an *E. coli* outbreak in the U.S. had occurred in 1982.

Pavia confirmed that the 1982 outbreak was, in fact, the first reported outbreak. But he assured Bill that HUS and *E. coli* O157:H7 had been on the scene much longer than that. Siegler had begun tracking cases in Utah starting in January 1971. He had the most comprehensive database on the subject in the U.S.

Pavia offered to send Bill a confidential, advance proof of the twenty-year study that he and Siegler planned to publish in the coming year. After reading it, Pavia suggested, Bill could get in touch with Siegler to go over the findings.

———

On January 29 Bill traveled to the Pierce County Courthouse in Tacoma and filed the suit. It accused Jack in the Box of negligently preparing, delivering, selling, and serving food unfit for human consumption. It also accused the restaurant chain of failing to observe Washington's minimum internal cooking temperatures for hamburger patties. The theory behind the suit was straightforward under Washington's Product Liability Act:

1. Hamburger is a product.

2. By virtue of being contaminated with *E. coli*, the product was faulty.

3. As the provider of the product, Jack in the Box was strictly liable for damages resulting from the faulty product it sold to customers.

There were also breach of warranty and negligence claims.

As soon as he left the courthouse, Bill called the media and briefed them on the suit. Bill was media savvy. In his four years of service on the Pullman City Council, he had gained an appreciation for the power of the press.

Shortly after he had taken office, he was commuting to work one morning on his motorcycle when he got broadsided by a big wheat truck. His bike got crushed and Bill was thrown more than fifty feet through the air before landing on the pavement and bouncing into a roadside ditch. ER doctors were amazed at being unable to detect any broken bones. But Bill had bruises everywhere . . . except his head, thanks to his helmet. When the press found out that the City Council's newest member had survived a potentially fatal motorcycle wreck, his picture ended up on the front page with an inspiring story that quoted him admonishing his constituents to always wear a helmet.

From that day forward, Bill had always stayed on a first-name basis with reporters. Generally, lawyers cling to the notion that talking to reporters is beneath them or unprofessional, but Bill saw the media as a multipurpose tool that could be used to speak to potential clients, exert pressure on an adversary, or create momentum toward changes in public policy. Like politicians, a lawyer doing personal-injury work was well served to make friends with those who bought ink by the barrel.

1

2

3

4

5

6   IN THE SUPERIOR COURT OF WASHINGTON FOR PIERCE COUNTY

7

8   KAREN GRAGG, as guardian ad litem   )   93 ˙2ʹ 00930 1
     of LORISSA GRAGG, a minor child,   )   NO.
9   individually and on behalf of   )
     themselves and all similarly   )
10   situated,   )   CLASS ACTION COMPLAINT
)   FOR DAMAGES
11   Plaintiffs,   )
)
12   v.   )
)   ﾟ﹒LED
13   FOODMAKER, INC., a Delaware   )   N ᴜᴏᴜNTY CLERK'S OFFICE
     corporation doing business as   )
14   "JACK-IN-THE-BOX" RESTAURANTS,   )   ˌM   ʲAN 2 9 1993 ᴩ﹒M﹒
)
15   Defendant.   )   ᴘᴵᴇᴦᴄᴇ ᴄᴏᴜɴᴛY ᴡᴀSʜINGᴛON
     ──────────────────────────────────   )

16

17   Plaintiffs, on behalf of themselves and all similarly

18   situated, for their claims against defendant, state and allege as

19   follows:

20   I. **PARTIES**

21   1. Plaintiff KAREN GRAGG, individually and as guardian ad

22   litem of LORISSA GRAGG, a minor child, is a resident of Pierce

23   County, Washington.

24   2. Defendant FOODMAKER, INC. is a Delaware corporation

25   doing business in Pierce County, Washington, and is the operator

26   of a nationwide chain of "Jack-In-The-Box" Restaurants which is

CLASS ACTION COMPLAINT - 1   KELLER ROHRBACK
N:\CLIENTS\20983\1\COMPLAIN   SUITE 3200
                                               1201 THIRD AVENUE
                                          SEATTLE, WASHINGTON 98101-3052
                                                 (206) 623-1900

Gragg v. Jack in the Box *was the first lawsuit filed by*
Bill Marler and his associates after the outbreak.

The day after Bill told the press about his suit against Jack in the Box, the phones started ringing at Keller Rohrback. Parents who had seen the press coverage of the firm's suit were calling for assistance. One by one they were connected with Bill, who began signing up new clients.

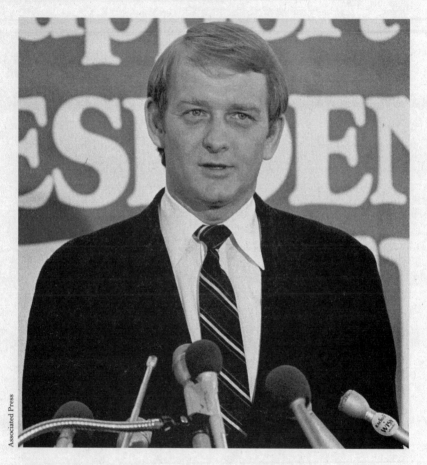

Jack in the Box hired President Jimmy Carter's former press secretary, Jody Powell, to guide CEO Bob Nugent through the public relations crisis.

12

TESTIMONY

SUZANNE KINER STARED AT THE DATE ON HER LITTLE POCKET CALENDAR: January 31. It was hard to believe that ten years earlier on this date she had given birth to Brianne. It was even harder to believe that Brianne wasn't awake to celebrate her tenth birthday. The two of them had now been at the hospital for over two weeks. Brianne had been in a coma for most of that time, and Suzanne hadn't left the building once. She rarely left Brianne's room. The nurses were starting to worry. Between the emotional stress and not eating, Suzanne had dropped almost forty pounds. A relative had to go out and buy her a couple of sweatshirts and some sweatpants because the clothes Suzanne had worn to the hospital no longer fit.

In spite of the circumstances, Suzanne was determined to make Brianne's birthday a memorable one. She had some decorations put up around the room and placed a Raggedy Ann doll above the bed. She also had a boom box brought in so she could play the song that Brianne's grammar school class had recorded for her. Balloons were tied to the bedrails.

After the celebration, Suzanne was once again alone with Brianne. She leaned over and whispered what she'd been telling her daughter for days. "This is a six-inch brick wall and you are four-foot eight inches high. It's your choice. All you have to do is step over the brick wall."

She'd convinced herself that if she kept saying it, the message would eventually get through.

The microbial data from the plants that were supplying meat to Vons had finally reached Dave Theno's desk. The results floored him. In all, Vons was getting its meat from eight different slaughter facilities scattered throughout the Midwest and the West. The internal testing done at these sites revealed that the amount of generic *E. coli* present in the raw meat was off the charts. Yet it had been shipped to Vons for processing, and then on to Jack in the Box for sale to its customers. And every one of these facilities was USDA inspected and approved.

Theno was convinced that in order for him to deliver the foolproof food-safety system that Nugent had requested, he'd have to recommend something far more radical than higher cooking temperatures and safer handling instructions for grill cooks. He had to develop a system that would get these slaughterhouses and meat-packing plants to clean up their act.

Meantime, Jack in the Box's PR team had a separate set of challenges. The outbreak had made it to the top of the network news. On February 1, Dan Rather, Tom Brokaw, and Peter Jennings all focused on *E. coli*. Officials at corporate headquarters watched anxiously as the most extensive report aired on ABC's *World News Tonight* with Peter Jennings.

"In Washington State," Jennings began, "the Jack in the Box fast-food chain has announced it will pay the hospital bills for the hundreds of customers who got sick after eating the company's hamburgers last month. The food poisoning epidemic involved a particularly virulent type of bacteria known as *E. coli*. It caused a great deal of anxiety. ABC's Judy Muller is in Seattle."

"Many of the critically ill victims," Judy Muller reported as children at a Seattle hospital appeared on screen behind her, "are children who experienced painful cramping, diarrhea, and, in some cases, temporary kidney failure that requires dialysis to cleanse the blood. Two children have died and dozens are hospitalized."

The report indicated that Jack in the Box restaurants had experienced a dramatic drop in business and some supermarkets had seen a 50 percent drop in hamburger-meat sales. But blame was also starting to shift to the USDA for its failure to adequately inspect America's beef supply. "There are many other inspectors who have contacted their hierarchy in the USDA and Food Safety Inspection Service and said, 'Hey, this ain't right out here,'" said one meat inspector. "But we're just not heard. And this is the result."

"Health officials agree," Judy Muller reported, "that thorough inspections at slaughterhouses and thorough cooking at restaurants are key to preventing a recurrence of this epidemic. Meanwhile, they recommend that Americans thoroughly wash their hands to prevent secondary infection and always order their hamburgers well done. Judy Muller, ABC News, Seattle."

"On Wall Street today," Peter Jennings said, "the Dow Jones Industrial Average rose more than 22 points to close at 3,332. The trading was heavy. In a moment—"

The PR team at Jack in the Box muted the TV. But they couldn't silence the relentless drumbeat of news coverage that was turning their restaurants into ghost towns. All they could do was cross their fingers and hope that Nugent's performance in front of Congress would not make matters worse.

Two Days Later
Wednesday, February 3, 1993
Washington, DC

It was early in the afternoon and Bob Nugent felt he was getting the runaround. He'd been to the offices of more than a dozen senators. All of them were on the subcommittee that would be questioning him the next day, and not one would meet with him. It angered Nugent that on the company's dime he'd flown all the way to DC at the senators' request, yet he couldn't get as much as a courtesy hello out of these guys.

A PR aide had made the trip to DC with Nugent. The aide had at least managed to arrange for a staffer on the subcommittee to give Nugent a walk-through on what to expect at the hearing. "This is the room you'll be in," the Senate committee staffer said, ushering Nugent and his aide inside.

Nugent looked at the dais where the senators would be seated. He could visualize the chairs occupied by men in suits, facing him.

"You'll be sitting at a table here," the staffer said, pointing. It was eye level with the dais. Nugent was relieved to see that his interrogators wouldn't be looking down on him.

"There will be a panel of four of you," the staffer continued. "And the committee will be asking questions of all four of you."

Nugent nodded. It all sounded pretty straightforward.

After the briefing, the PR aide suggested knocking on a few more senators' doors, but Nugent wanted none of it. Besides, he couldn't wait to get away from his PR aide. His youth and high-strung personality had been grating on Nugent's nerves all day. The guy worked for a PR firm in LA that had been hired by Jack in the Box's insurance carrier. Nugent thought the insurance company was wasting its money. He told his aide he'd meet him back at the hotel later that afternoon. It was a polite way of saying, "Get lost."

Finally alone, Nugent headed off to a private meeting with Jody Powell & Associates, the highly respected Washington PR firm established by President Jimmy Carter's former press secretary. A friend of Nugent's had arranged for him to meet with an associate there. When Nugent arrived, he was shown into a conference room, where sandwiches and beverages were arranged on the table. Hardly in the mood to eat, Nugent just sat there until the door opened and a man walked in.

"Hi, I'm Jody Powell," he said, extending his hand.

Surprised, Nugent stood up and introduced himself. He had not expected to meet Powell himself. "I was introduced to your firm by a friend," Nugent said. "My friend knows—"

"Yeah, I know," Powell said. "She should be in here in a minute."

Powell invited Nugent to sit down and get comfortable. The two men started talking shop, and they hit it off quickly. "Why don't you tell me what's going on?" Powell said.

"I'm in deep shit here, Jody," Nugent began, telling him about the testimony he was scheduled to deliver before the Senate. "And I have a PR firm that I'm working with, and I don't have any confidence in them."

Powell nodded.

"To give you an example of why I don't have any confidence in the firm, this is the damn six-minute opening remarks that were developed for me by the firm," Nugent said, waving the document in his hand. "It's just horrible."

Powell asked to take a look at it, and Nugent pushed it across the table. After a quick read, Powell shoved it back. "I agree with you," Powell said.

Then Powell talked about the whole business of congressional hearings. He had a folksy style, but it was immediately clear that he knew his way around trouble. When he was press secretary, the Carter White House had had one crisis after another: a crippling energy crisis that produced massive lines at gas pumps, the invasion of Afghanistan by the Soviet Union, the Iran hostage crisis, and finally a failed hostage-rescue attempt. Powell had had to face the cameras for each of these episodes. Jack in the Box was a huge nightmare to Nugent, but to Powell it was just another passing storm. For the first time since the start of the outbreak, Nugent felt confident around someone who did PR.

"Would your firm be interested in helping me?" Nugent asked.

"*I'll* do it," Powell said.

Nugent was pleasantly surprised at that. By this point, the woman he was supposed to meet with had entered the room. Polite and competent, she handed her business card to Nugent and said he could call on her any time.

Nugent told Powell and his associate that he needed to call back to San Diego and get approval to fire the LA PR firm and hire Powell. He was confident it could all be worked out by morning.

Before Nugent left, Powell made a copy of the six-minute opening statement prepared for Nugent by the other firm.

Later that evening Nugent rejoined his PR aide, who had arranged for an ex-congressman to put Nugent through a mock Senate hearing. The simulated question-and-answer session was staged at a television studio not far from Capitol Hill. Nugent's lawyer, Fred Gordon, attended the session, too. He had flown in from San Diego to accompany Nugent to the hearing. After nearly three hours of questioning, Nugent was exhausted and his head was pounding. He'd had enough.

It was 10:00 p.m. when Gordon and Nugent arrived back at the Mayflower Hotel. Nugent checked his messages at the main lobby desk. The attendant handed him an oversized manila envelope. Declining Gordon's invitation to get a nightcap, Nugent retreated to his room and opened the parcel. It contained a revamped six-minute opening statement for his congressional testimony, written personally by Jody Powell.

Nugent sank into a soft chair and read it. "Much, much better," he said to himself after working his way through the document. He undressed, turned out the lights, and got into bed.

Still on West Coast time, Fred Gordon turned on the television and started channel surfing. He ended up watching ABC's *PrimeTime Live*. Anchor Sam Donaldson was talking about an undercover investigation into meat-packing plants that the show had done a year earlier. "Little did we realize how soon that report by John Quiñones would come back to haunt us," Donaldson said as the program cut to a USDA meat inspector from nine months earlier.

"I predict," the inspector said, "that you will see more cases of food poisoning, people dying, and people getting sick from eating contaminated meat."

"That warning," correspondent John Quiñones said, "issued on our program nine months ago was all too prophetic. In the last three weeks nearly five hundred people who ate hamburgers at Jack in the Box restaurants in Washington, Oregon, Idaho, Nevada, and California have come down with severe food poisoning. Two children have died, over a hundred others have been hospitalized."[*]

Gordon couldn't believe what he was seeing.

Then the report cut to a hidden camera. "When *PrimeTime* went undercover at four slaughterhouses last May we discovered how easy it is for meat to get contaminated and get by inspectors undetected. Our hidden cameras captured entire carcasses falling on floors covered with cow feces, urine, and blood, only to be hung back on production lines where the tainted meat contaminated other carcasses. Some of the dirty beef was picked up off the floor and loaded directly onto trucks for delivery to grocery stores and restaurants throughout the country."

A USDA inspector then admitted that this sort of thing went on every day.

---

[*]The death of Lauren Rudolph in San Diego had not at this point been officially associated with the outbreak; the two deaths in Seattle, of Michael Nole and Celina Shribbs, had been determined to be a result of the outbreak.

By the end of the report, Gordon was livid. He shut off the TV and went to bed.

———————

Tossing and turning, Nugent finally sat up in bed and looked at the clock: 2:00 a.m.. Unable to stop worrying about his testimony, he got out of bed, turned on the lamp, and reached for a pad and a pen. He still wasn't completely satisfied with his opening statement. Using Powell's much-improved draft as a guide; he attempted to rewrite it in longhand, hoping to personalize it.

Before he knew it, his mind drifted to his two daughters, ages twenty-three and twenty-four. They were beautiful and smart and educated. But he remembered when they had been little and innocent and carefree. Then he thought about the fact that he was leading a company that sold a product that had killed three children that were little and innocent and carefree. After twenty-five years in the food industry, he suddenly looked at his occupation—this business of food—in a whole different light. All alone in a dimly lit hotel room, he began to cry. *God, I've got to get a hold of myself,* he told himself, wiping his eyes.

Two hours later he finished writing. It was 4:00 a.m., and he realized he had a problem. *How in the hell and am I going to get this thing typed up?*

He grabbed a couple of hours of sleep before he pulled out the business card of Jody Powell's associate. At 6:00 a.m. he called her, and she dispatched someone to the Mayflower, assuring Nugent that they'd type his remarks, have seventy-five copies made, and get them distributed to the committee members before the hearing.

Relieved, Nugent picked up the *New York Times.* His anxiety immediately returned when he saw the headline "Jack in the Box's Worst Nightmare."

"Since the outbreak of food poisoning from hamburger sold at Jack in the Box outlets here in mid-January left two children dead, the stock of the chain's parent company, Foodmaker, Inc., has dropped more than 30 percent," the story began. Then came a quote from Nugent: "In the last 10 years, we've sold 400 million pounds of hamburger safely and without incident. Then bang, it hits you. It's your worst, worst nightmare."

Nugent's blood began to boil when he read the next paragraph. "Meanwhile, the United States Agriculture Department and state health officials say the bacteria could have been killed if Jack in the Box had cooked the hamburger at 155 degrees as required by the state. . . . Analysts worry whether Jack in the Box will be able to recover."

By the time Nugent met Gordon for breakfast on the main floor of the hotel at 7:30 a.m., both were livid. Gordon complained about the *PrimeTime Live* segment on the unsanitary conditions at U.S. slaughterhouses.

"*These* are the type of places we're getting meat from and the government is blaming *us* for not cooking it?" Nugent said in disgust.

When the two men arrived at the Capitol, they tracked down the staffer that had given Nugent a brief tour of the hearing room the previous day. "There's been a change in plans," the staffer told them.

Nugent gave Gordon a disgusted look. He hated surprises like this.

The staffer led them down a hallway toward a different hearing room. It was easy to find. TV cameras and reporters congregated outside the doors. Nugent brushed past them and looked inside. The new hearing room was much larger. And the seats for the Senate committee members were elevated above the witness table.

"There's been one other change," the committee staffer told Nugent. "Instead of being on a panel with three other witnesses, you'll be testifying alone." Then the Senate staffer walked off.

Nugent felt like he was being set up. Gordon agreed.

It was 10:34 a.m. when Senator Tom Daschle called the hearing to order. "We hope to examine the extent of the problem our nation faces from *E. coli* O157:H7 and what changes to federal food-inspection programs should be made to ensure safe meat for American consumers," he began. "For the good of our children and the confidence of their families, we must continue to have the safest food supply in the world."

Daschle pointed out that two children had already died after eating a Jack in the Box hamburger. And a number of other children, including Brianne Kiner remained in critical condition at Children's Hospital in Seattle. Then he praised President Bill Clinton for promptly dispatching Secretary of Agriculture Michael Espy to Seattle right after the start of the outbreak.

"Before calling on the Secretary for his testimony, let me ask my colleagues if they have any opening statements they would care to make."

Senator Patrick Leahy spoke first. "Thank you, Mr. Chairman, and I commend you and your ranking member and those who are holding this hearing. I think it is extremely valuable. I want to state publicly what I said privately in a meeting earlier this morning with Secretary Espy. I told him that I wanted to commend him for the way he is handling this outbreak of foodborne illness."

Nugent knew one thing. Secretary Espy didn't have any trouble getting a one-on-one meeting with the senator. Listening to Leahy heap praise on his fellow politicians, Nugent couldn't help getting a little jaded. These guys were ultimately responsible for the laws and regulations governing America's food safety. Yet they were caught flat-footed by *E. coli* and they'd been asleep at the switch while the conditions at U.S. slaughterhouses had gotten more and more lax.

"Mr. Secretary," Leahy continued, "it occurred four days before you were sworn in as Secretary. You became Secretary; you immediately flew to Washington State to look into it yourself. It sends a powerful message, and I know you intend to offer a plan to help prevent these types of outbreaks in the future."

It was all Nugent could do not to roll his eyes.

Secretary Espy kept his testimony brief, pointing out that he'd been on the job only fifteen days and acknowledging the obvious—that the government's inspection system was no longer adequate, something he vowed to change.

After Espy concluded and stepped away from the witness table, Daschle called Nugent. He took his place at the table, stated his name and title for the record, and expressed appreciation for the opportunity to appear.

"A number of people, mostly children, recently became ill after eating contaminated meat at some of our restaurants," Nugent began. "Tragically, two have died and two remain in critical condition. Words cannot express my sorrow or the sadness of our employees. Our hearts ache for the families and the friends of the young boys who died and we pray for the recovery of those who are still ill. There is always much soul-searching after such a tragedy, but we recognize that no amount of reflection can minimize the pain or undo the loss."

These were the words that he had penned hours earlier in his hotel room. After speaking from the heart, he made the points he had come to Washington to make.

"But it is important to note that the contaminated meat that was infected with the *E. coli* O157:H7 bacteria before delivery to our restaurants had passed all USDA inspections. Every one of our chefs had carefully followed all federal food-preparation standards.

"In fact, I just recently learned that the Centers for Disease Control reports that some twenty thousand cases of infection from *E. coli* O157:H7 occur every year, and every year some of these outbreaks are traceable to contaminated food that is served in restaurants, hospitals, and other institutions. Clearly, the current USDA meat-inspection system and federal food preparation standards are not providing the protection Americans deserve."

Nugent had wasted no time before pointing the finger at the senators. They were the ones that had oversight of the USDA.

"Thank you very much, Mr. Nugent, for your opening remarks," Daschle said. "You have noted publicly that Jack in the Box was not cooking its meat in compliance with Washington State standards. . . . Is that an accurate understanding of the situation?"

"Mr. Chairman, the cooking procedures that we have established and have been in place for many, many years, at least since 1976, were designed to ensure that the internal cooking temperature of our hamburger patties was 140 degrees."

"Is the Washington State standard 155?" Daschle asked.

"Yes, it is."

"So you were below the Washington State standard."

"Correct."

Seated behind Nugent, Gordon didn't like where this was headed.

"What temperature are you frying your food today?" Daschle continued.

"The internal temperature of the hamburgers," Nugent said, ". . . now exceeds 163 degrees."

Idaho senator Larry Craig wanted to know if Jack in the Box's grills had a timing mechanism to tell cooks when a patty was done.

"Yes," Nugent said. Cooks hit a button when the patty was placed on the grill. A timer would go off, telling the cook when to flip the burger and again when the burger was fully cooked. Then the cook was supposed to make a visual inspection for any pink and to ensure that the meat juices were coming out clear.

Craig asked if the line grill cooks were an integral part of the process for cooking hamburgers.

Nugent confirmed that they were.

Daschle wanted to get back to the 155-degree cooking standard in Washington. "Why was it not the policy of the company to have a range of temperatures that exceeded 155 to ensure that pathogens such as this would not be present in the food consumed?" he asked.

"The cooking procedures that were in place at the time of the incident did comply with the federal regulation of 140," Nugent said.

"You were not aware of the Washington State regulation of 155?" Daschle asked.

"We were not aware of the Washington State regulation."

Fred Gordon cringed. It drove him nuts every time Nugent used the pronoun *we*. It was one thing to say "I" didn't know. Chief executives of national corporations aren't expected to have personal knowledge of intricate details of state regulations. But those responsible for implementing the regulations are. And by saying "we," Nugent was admitting that the company had violated the law in Washington. That was not a good thing to say when children were dead. When they got back to San Diego, Gordon planned to tell Nugent in no uncertain terms that he had to change what he was saying or say nothing at all.

Washington senator Patty Murray picked up where Craig and Daschle left off. "It seems to me," she said, "that the temperature of the patty depends, as you have said, on the burner heat as well as the time that you flip it over and a visual inspection. So that tells me that your employee is very integral to the safety of the individual hamburger. Those employees—how do you train them?"

Nugent said they received video training, written instructions, and on-the-job training by managers. Also, a new step had been added as a result of the outbreak: "Simply probe the inside of the patty to ensure that there is no pink and that the juices coming through are clear," he said.

"The chef, then, is responsible for doing that, correct?" Murray asked.

"Correct."

"The chefs in your restaurants, are there any of them that are sixteen- or seventeen-year-olds?"

"There are some that are sixteen and seventeen."

"So they are directly responsible for doing that last visual check?"

"They are responsible for performing the function, yes."

The implication was obvious. Something as serious as making sure that ground beef was cooked sufficiently to kill pathogens had been put in the hands of teenagers. Nugent was beside himself. The line of questioning was a remarkable blend of arrogance and ignorance. Had any of these senators set foot in a McDonald's anytime in the past, oh, twenty years? Were they unaware that teenagers were a sizable chunk of the work force in the fast-food industry? And did they not know that teenagers cooked and handled the food? It wasn't as if the situation in Jack in the Box kitchens were new or unique. They mirrored the industry.

"Mr. Nugent," Senator Daschle interjected, "let me just follow up one more time because I am most troubled by the practices, and I don't mean to single you out." He asked why the technical staff at Jack in the Box hadn't come to their own conclusion about the need to cook beef to a higher temperature in order to kill *E. coli*.

The question galled Nugent. "For forty-two years we've had a system for cooking that has enabled us to serve safe, wholesome, and good quality products to hundreds of millions of customers. We have served hundreds of millions of hamburgers, and we constantly are evaluating those procedures to ensure that we are meeting our obligations to our customers and public safety." Then he turned the tables on Daschle. "Historically, we have relied upon the government and our suppliers to provide us any information that would suggest that we need to make adjustments in our standards."

Daschle pointed out that the state government had in fact provided Jack in the Box with information notifying them that their meat should be cooked to 155 degrees. "I underscore what you have just said about your record," Daschle said. "It is commendable . . . but obviously it only takes one case like this to destroy an otherwise impeccable record."

Daschle paused before continuing. "I guess I am just curious as to what goes through the minds of those executives making decisions like this when it comes to something as important as this, that is, the standards that must be set to ensure adequate confidence about the reliability of the products they are serving."

Nugent wanted to call Daschle a pompous ass, but he held his tongue. "Mr. Chairman," he said in exasperation, "I wish I had known about the Washington State regulation in May of 1992 when it was established. . . . I wish I would have known about the outbreak in Walla Walla where there were two deaths in 1986. I didn't.

"I have instituted a full-scale investigation. We are pulling records from all of our restaurants. We are interviewing all of our employees to find who knew what and, if anybody knew anything, why didn't our corporate headquarters know it? At this point, all I can tell you is that I didn't know it. I wish I had."

"Well, again, Mr. Nugent," Daschle said, "we are very pleased that you could share your experiences and your thoughts with us this morning. I don't know what your schedule is, but if it would allow for you to stay for the rest of the hearing in order to return to the table at the end, I would appreciate it."

Nugent gathered up his notes and stepped away from the witness table. Gordon was waiting for him. "Fat chance in hell I'm hanging around," he told Gordon. "Get me the f—— out of this town."

Reporters shoved cameras and tape recorders in Nugent's face as Gordon whisked him through the hall, out the door, and into a car waiting outside.

"Why'd they even bring me here?" Nugent complained. "They had zero interest in what I was saying."

All the way to the airport, both men vented. "Of course," Gordon said, "no one gets to ask them the question: 'Well, what the f—— have you done lately?' 'Why haven't you required beef processors to even test?' 'Why don't you require them to even clean the shit off the cows before they bring them into the slaughterhouses?'"

Nugent couldn't get over the senators' duplicity. They'd go hard after a restaurant serving the food. But they were silent on the industrial farms, slaughterhouses, and meat-packing plants that supplied the food to the restaurants. That was because the politicians would have to acknowledge that the USDA had such an abysmal record when it came to letting contaminated meat into the stream of commerce.

"It's a joke," Gordon explained. "The reality is that if a slaughterhouse gets caught by a USDA inspector, the place is *really* a piece of shit. These inspectors are never there. When they *are* there, they've got two people watching six thousand cows per day get slaughtered. That's bullshit!"

13

EXPERT WITNESSES

When Bill received the promised materials from Dr. Andrew Pavia at the University of Utah's medical school, he carefully studied the preliminary findings from the landmark study. It pointed out that HUS had been an important public-health problem in Utah for twenty years and about 90 percent of childhood cases occurred after bloody diarrhea. The evidence implicating *E. coli* O157:H7 as the primary cause of HUS was mounting.

After going through the report, Bill called the medical school again. This time he reached Siegler at his desk. They struck up a friendly tone right off the bat. Siegler shared the cartoon that he had tacked up over his desk. It showed the Jack in the Box logo above the words "We're cooking the shit out of our hamburgers."

Bill shared Siegler's sense of humor but quickly moved to the outbreak.

Siegler assured him that a large-scale outbreak like the one in Seattle had been building for years. He told Bill about a recent experience when he'd taken his wife to a fast-food restaurant in Salt Lake City. She had ordered a hamburger that was red in the middle. Siegler took the undercooked burger to the restaurant manager. "See this?" Siegler told him. "This is the kind of hamburger that kills my patients."

Siegler said his wife's experience was indicative of a large-scale problem. "There really aren't uniform regulations about cooking ground beef," Siegler explained. "Unfortunately, cooking until the meat looks brown and the juices are running clear doesn't necessarily mean that you've reached the temperature required to kill *E. coli.*"

Bill had had no idea.

Previously frozen burger patties, Siegler explained, can often look brown even before they are sufficiently cooked.

Bill always took notes when talking to experts. But as he listened to Siegler he made a mental note to himself—*no hamburgers for Morgan.*

After Bill brought Siegler up to speed on the situation in Seattle, Siegler told Bill that the Seattle area was fortunate to have a guy like Dr. Phil Tarr at Children's Hospital at the time of the outbreak. He probably knew more about the formation of *E. coli* and what it did to children than anyone in pediatric medicine.

Bill wondered what the difference was between Siegler and Tarr in terms of their research into *E. coli.*

"We both have a pretty keen interest in the subject," Siegler explained. "Phil Tarr's is through the GI tract. He's a gastroenterologist. I'm a nephrologist. My angle is the kidney. I get involved because of hemolytic-uremic syndrome. *Uremic* means kidney failure."

Bill liked the way Siegler simplified things. He had a natural way of teaching while he talked, making complex things understandable. Those were the attributes of a good expert witness.

Bill said he was looking to get a better understanding of HUS.

"Only about 10 percent of those who get *E. coli* and get diarrhea go on to get HUS," Siegler explained. "It's probably because the number of receptors varies from person to person. They are in the small blood vessels of the intestines. Then they bleed into the diarrhea."

Bill told Siegler that he had talked to Pavia and had been briefed on the twenty-year study they'd been working on.

It is clear, Siegler said, that about 90 percent of the HUS cases in children occurred after diarrhea that was typically bloody. And *E. coli* O157:H7 was emerging as the primary cause.

Bill knew he had the right guy. He asked Siegler about becoming an expert witness—someone he could call on to guide him through the literature and help explain the syndrome.

In all his years in medicine, Siegler had never served as an expert witness and he'd never testified in court proceedings. To his knowledge there had never been any lawsuits associated with *E. coli* and HUS. But things were changing. Children were dying and *E. coli* had clearly taken center stage as a foodborne illness in one of America's most popular food items—hamburgers. Siegler agreed to be Bill's expert witness. And Pavia signed on to work with Bill, too.

As soon as Bob Nugent got back to San Diego, the company's corporate communications office got inundated with requests from news agencies and television programs. Most of them wanted to interview Nugent. Even Phil Donahue had planned a show around the *E. coli* outbreak.

The first thing Nugent did was fire the company's outside PR firm. Then he hired Jody Powell, who flew out from Washington right away. One of the immediate issues to resolve was how to deal with the question that kept coming up at the hearing: Had the company known about the 155-degree rule in Washington? The answer had tremendous legal and political implications. Powell sat in on a meeting between Gordon and Nugent over how to handle the situation. Emotions quickly got the best of them, especially when Gordon told Nugent to stop saying "we" didn't know.

"I don't want you saying that," Gordon said.

"But damn it, Fred, it's the truth."

"Bob, I don't give a damn!"

Gordon had just filed the lawsuit against Vons. He knew Vons's defense would be that Jack in the Box had been negligent in its handling and cooking procedures. "If you want to destroy our case now, go ahead," Gordon told Nugent.

Nugent was sick and tired of lawyers and PR people telling him what to say and what not to say. Facts were facts. He hadn't known about the damn regulation in Washington.

"Bob," Gordon yelled, "if you don't know what the law is, why in hell would you run around and admit that? Why would you keep saying it?"

Nugent had more to think about than one lawsuit. He was trying to save a company. The biggest problem the company had was credibility amongst its customers. Lying at this point wasn't going to help.

Gordon laughed out of frustration. He knew that Ken Dunkley had said he hadn't known about the regulation. But Gordon had a hard time believing that the company hadn't been notified of the regulation change. In his mind it was only a matter of time before the ongoing internal investigation turned up proof that the state had notified the company. Regardless, Nugent's answer compromised the company legally.

"It doesn't matter if you didn't know," Gordon shouted. "If you are a company doing business in a state that has a law and you come out and say we didn't know, well, you are deemed to have known! And you should have known! So saying we didn't know hurts! It doesn't help!"

San Diego attorney Fred Gordon represented Jack in the Box in a lawsuit against its meat supplier.

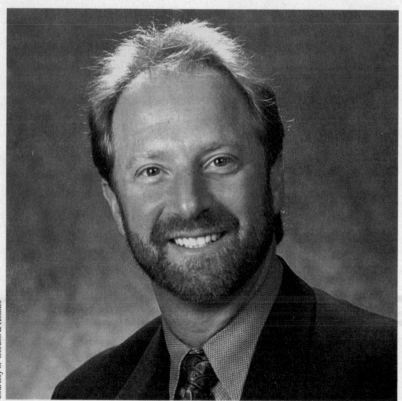

Gordon stormed out.

Nugent looked at Powell. "He's basically saying don't admit to anything," Nugent said.

Powell nodded in agreement.

"I'm saying we have to tell the truth."

Powell nodded again.

"What would you do?" Nugent asked.

"I'd tell the lawyer to shove it up his ass," Powell said.

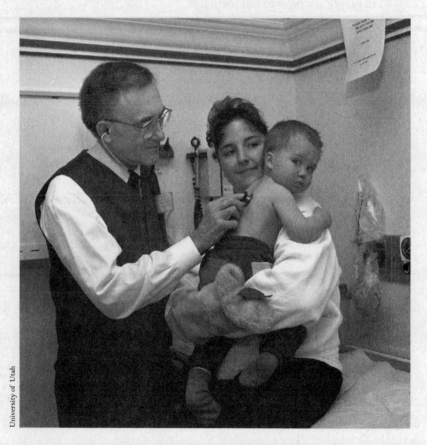

Attorney Bill Marler hired Salt Lake City physician Richard Siegler, a leading national authority on kidney disease in children, as an expert witness in the suits against Jack in the Box.

14

NO MIRACLES OR TRAGEDIES

In his brief foray into politics, Bill had learned the importance of knowing more than your opponents. Politicians have to be familiar with a wide range of topics and issues. Lawyers are in the same boat. They have to become experts on whatever subject is at the heart of a case. To become an expert on *E. coli*, Bill spent as much time as possible talking to doctors and microbiologists. One thing that intrigued him was the notion that a child who hadn't eaten contaminated hamburger meat could nonetheless die from *E. coli*. On February 20, seventeen-month-old Riley Detwiler died from *E. coli* poisoning at Children's Hospital despite not having eaten ground beef. Rather, Riley had contracted the disease by coming in contact with another sick child at a day care center. Riley was the fourth fatality of the outbreak. Bill called Siegler for an explanation.

It impressed Siegler that a lawyer was so interested in the science behind the disease. In the case of *E. coli*, there were lots of mysteries still to be cracked. "I've got quite a few horror stories," Siegler said. He shared one of his tragic cases from Idaho that involved two toddlers who lived across the street from each other. Their mothers were close friends and sometimes bathed their two-year-olds together. One of the two-year-olds got diarrhea. The mothers didn't think much about its being contagious. "The kid across the street bathed with the one that had diarrhea," Siegler said. "The kid across the street got severe diarrhea and got HUS and died. The kid who gave it to him survived."

A couple of years earlier, a sixteen-month old boy from rural Idaho had developed a respiratory infection and been treated with amoxicillin. The next day the boy began vomiting and developed severe diarrhea that left him dehydrated. He was transferred from a hospital in Idaho to University of Utah Hospital after suffering two seizures in one day. Stool cultures confirmed the presence of *E. coli* O157:H7. But a case study turned up no direct evidence that the infant had eaten anything contaminated with *E. coli*. Nor did the boy attend a day care facility where germs could have been passed. However, the infant's father worked on a dairy farm. Fecal specimens were collected from the sixty dairy cattle at the farm and subsequently frozen and sent to the CDC for examination. Isolates confirmed the presence of *E. coli* O157:H7.

"This organism inhabits the intestines of dairy cattle and is a frequent cause of diarrhea (often bloody) and HUS in North America," Siegler wrote at the time. "Recognized risk factors for *E. coli* O157:H7 infection includes eating inadequately cooked ground beef, drinking unpasteurized milk, person to person contact, as may occur in families and in children attending day-care centers."

Siegler suspected that in this case the father had transmitted the infection to the infant. The most likely culprit was his work boots, which carried manure on the soles. The father had worn the boots across an area of the floor where the infant typically crawled. If the child crawled where the father had walked, the *E. coli* would have easily transferred via hand to mouth.

The more Bill learned about *E. coli* the more he started to adjust his eating habits. He'd already told Julie that their daughter, Morgan, should never be allowed to eat hamburger. Now he was adding unpasteurized milk to the Off Limits list.

———

When Brianne slipped into a coma, Suzanne's older brother, Garry Hubert, had flown up from San Francisco to offer moral support and legal advice to his sister. A successful lawyer at a Bay-area firm, Hubert specialized in insurance law. One look at Brianne convinced him that Suzanne and her family were going to need help navigating through all the insurance and liability issues raised by the *E. coli* poisoning.

Eventually, the family would have to contend with Jack in the Box over damages. In the meantime, Hubert wanted everything carefully documented. But the last thing Hubert wanted to do was give his sister one more thing to worry about. Instead, he promised he'd handle all the legal work. The first thing he did was look for a top-notch private security firm that had experience with corporate litigation. After doing a little research, he settled on Trident Investigative Service, Inc., a Seattle firm run by a private investigator named Mike Canaan.

Canaan's path to becoming a PI had not been typical. When Jimmy Carter was president, Canaan was a U.S. Marine assigned to the presidential helicopter based at Quantico, Virginia. After a distinguished career in the marines, he went into law enforcement until entering the private sector and opening his own firm doing specialized investigatory work for law firms, insurance companies, and big corporations involved in litigation. When Canaan got the call from Garry Hubert, he knew the assignment was not the norm. But he viewed the chance to help Brianne Kiner as an honor. Like everyone else in Seattle, he'd been following her case through the media. He signed a confidentiality agreement with Hubert and immediately paid a visit to the hospital to meet the family.

With a military background and a career in law enforcement, Canaan had seen a lot. But he struggled the first time he saw Brianne, lying there comatose and naked other than some bandages over her pubic area, her mouth propped open by a breathing tube. A wide incision ran from her collar bone to her pubic bone. Her organs were so swollen that doctors were unable to suture her shut after surgery. Instead, they covered the area in gauze, which was absorbing body fluids and secretions.

To Canaan, the sight of Brianne in that state was the best evidence of what *E. coli* had done to her. He suggested to Garry and Suzanne that they allow him to photograph Brianne's injuries as evidence. They both agreed, and Canaan promised to put that task on the top of his To Do list.

Dave Theno had promised to deliver Bob Nugent a plan to overhaul the company's food-safety protocols within thirty days. Ahead of schedule, he requested an opportunity to make a presentation to Nugent and other senior executives.

He began by introducing them to a new acronym: HACCP (pronounced "hass-ip"), the abbreviation for Hazard Analysis and Critical Control Point, a system geared for analyzing hazards at critical points along the food production chain.

"There are points in your production process that have the most risk," Theno explained. "And you have to control them. So HACCP is a process-control system that basically manages food safety by managing the 10 points that control 90 percent of the outcome. It's the 90-10 rule."

Nugent asked the origins of HACCP.

Theno gave him the background. The system had first been developed by Pillsbury for NASA, which wanted a way to insure that the astronauts didn't get food poisoning in space. That meant guaranteeing that the food was grown, processed, and packaged in a manner that was free of pathogens. The National Academy of Sciences, a group that makes recommendations to the FDA and USDA on cutting-edge food-safety threats, subsequently recommended taking portions of the HACCP system for astronauts and adopting it for some food products sold to consumers. So in 1985 both agencies jointly recommended HACCP as the most effective strategy for controlling pathogenic bacteria, such as *E. coli*, in precooked, ready-to-eat food products available in grocery stores.

"Is this system being used in beef plants?" Nugent asked.

"Not yet," Theno said. "Everyone says HACCP can't work in fresh meat."

Theno, however, believed otherwise. And he told the group that one of his previous clients—one of the largest poultry producers in the U.S.—had had him set up a HACCP system to counter *Salmonella* in chickens.

Nugent asked the results.

"We drove *Salmonella* down to zero," Theno said.

Nugent raised his eyebrows and asked what a HACCP system would look like in a beef operation.

Theno was already headed there. He told the group that there would be four basic components to the process:

1. Raw Materials (the meat): Selecting the right beef suppliers.

2. Distribution (transportation): Protecting food products en route from the manufacturer to the restaurants.

3. Restaurant Safety: A set of safety checks for restaurant handlers.

4. Corporate Infrastructure: Training programs for employees and incentives that motivate employees to follow the programs.

Theno had no doubt that the company could accomplish the third and fourth stages, since those applied exclusively to what went on in Jack in the Box restaurants, where the company had more direct control. The first two components, on the other hand, had much more to do with Jack in the Box's business partners, such beef cattle farmers, slaughterhouses, meat processors, and meat distributors. They would be much harder to control and monitor. So Theno spent more time explaining what it would take to insure that the restaurant was getting a safe product.

He had devised a HACCP safety checklist for beef slaughterhouses. It spelled out best practices for skinning animals, washing carcasses, eviscerating the carcass without breaking the intestines (where *E. coli* is stored), washing and administering bacteria treatments to the raw product, and then storing and fabricating the carcasses. Then he had a separate safety checklist for the meat-grinding and patty-making facilities—the middlemen between the slaughterhouses and Jack in the Box.

The big thing, he pointed out, was the presence of microbial profiling of the meat at key stages in the process. Under Theno's plan, all future beef suppliers for Jack in the Box would have to furnish a microbial profile that would certify the absence of harmful levels of pathogens in the product.

"Remember," Theno said, "HACCP is farm-to-fork. So you have to control the whole process. You can't have areas where miracles or tragedies happen."

Hands shot up around the room. More than one member of the group pointed out that none of their suppliers or the slaughterhouses were doing this kind of testing.

Theno acknowledged this wouldn't be easy. "I'm not too sure everyone will do this sampling," he said. "Jack in the Box has to find people that will sample beef."

As Nugent listened, he realized that what Theno was describing was truly revolutionary. The food industry had become organized in a way where no one was accountable for the integrity of the finished product except the guy who sold directly to the consumer. A rancher who raised cattle was free of responsibility once he handed the cow off to the feedlot. Once the feedlot owners loaded the cows onto trucks headed for the slaughterhouse, the feedlot owners were no longer responsible. The same held true for the slaughterhouse operators once they handed the raw meat off to the processing and packing plants. And on and on it went. Food purveyors like Jack in the Box, never mind the consumer who actually ate the food, had no idea where the raw materials had come from or whether or not they were processed safely. The *E. coli* outbreak in Seattle was a manifestation of the flaws in that model. Theno was proposing a system that would enable Jack in the Box to control every step of the process.

"What this program does," Theno reiterated, "is allow us to profile suppliers and select the ones that are doing a good job of microbial control."

Someone had a question about component number three, which entailed overhauling handling and cooking procedures in all 1,155 Jack in the Box restaurants.

This, Theno acknowledged, would be a big undertaking that would entail retraining thousands of employees on all sorts of new techniques, from using tongs to handle hamburger patties to installing antimicrobial soap dispensers in restaurants. "But if you control the threats behind you," Theno pointed out, "the restaurant level is easier."

Nugent wanted to know more about the fourth component, what Theno called the corporate programs.

Theno said the corporate programs essentially involved incentives to motivate employees to follow the new rules. Whereas just about any other screwup in the restaurant business was resolved with a modest amount of money, "if you screw up food safety," Theno said, "you bet your business. It's that simple."

Nobody could argue with that.

When the meeting broke up, Nugent called Theno into his office. "Dave," he said, "we'd like to hire you to implement this plan."

"You mean as a consultant, right?"

"No, no. We'd like to hire you to do this full-time. We think we need you full-time."

"Ah . . . Bob, you know, that's very flattering, but . . ."

Theno wasn't sure what to say next. He knew what he was thinking. *I've got a private consulting company that's doing so well that it's practically printing money. Jack in the Box just blew up the food-safety world. And last I checked, your stock is at three dollars a share and the banks might foreclose on you. And I'm going to give up my business to come and work here full-time? No thanks.*

But he was more tactful with Nugent. "Bob, I don't mean to be harsh. But you guys have some issues here."

Nugent laughed. "We know. But our people know you. They like you. We think you'd be good for us and we'd be good for you."

Theno knew one thing—he really liked Nugent and his approach. He'd been around a lot of executives in the food industry, and none of them seemed to care about food safety the way Nugent did.

"Bob let me think about this," he said. "You understand my dilemma."

"Of course," Nugent said. "Think about it."

February 23, 1993

Suzanne Kiner felt like death was tapping her on the shoulder. Brianne had been comatose for five weeks without improvement. The hospital had been gently coaxing Suzanne toward the decision to remove Brianne from the life-support system. In her mind, Suzanne had been running through the questions that come with planning a funeral. She wondered about the burial site. *It needs to be a beautiful cemetery,* she thought. But is has to be one that I don't drive past every day.

Then there was the question of what to bury Brianne in. *The prom dress she'll never get to wear?* she wondered. *Or maybe it should be the wedding gown she'll never get to wear. Perhaps it should just be her favorite rumpled-up, pink jogging suit.*

There were just too many choices. Overwhelmed, Suzanne left the hospital and slipped into a nearby Catholic Church to pray. As she knelt in a middle pew, she overheard two women in the pew behind her.

"I don't think that Kiner girl is going to make it," one whispered to the other.

Suzanne slowly turned around, her lips quivering and tears streaming down her face. "That's my daughter you are talking about," she whispered. "That's my daughter."

Embarrassed, the women apologized while another woman beside Suzanne grabbed her trembling hand. "I'm praying for your daughter," the woman said.

Back at the hospital Suzanne entered Brianne's room hoping for a miracle. But Brianne's brain wave remained flat on the screen of the electroencephalograph, forcing Suzanne to come to grips with the cold reality that her daughter's medical hurdles were a lot higher than a six-inch brick wall. Desperate, she turned to a few vials of holy water that had been given to her by women of faith—complete strangers. Suzanne often wondered whether the stuff had any real power. But she didn't doubt the power of positive thinking.

Looking around and seeing no nurses in sight, Suzanne removed the tops of the vials and poured the contents all over Brianne's head. She even put a few drops in Brianne's IV. *This is it*, she thought. *I can't beg any more time for her.*

It was almost midnight, which would mark the start of Ash Wednesday.

15

THE AWAKENING

BILL WASN'T PLEASED WHEN HE GOT WORD THAT JACK IN THE BOX had filed a motion to remove his class-action suit from state court in Tacoma to federal court. In a case against an out-of-town corporation, the last place Bill wanted to be was in federal court. For starters, things moved much more slowly there. It wasn't uncommon in situations like this for a year to go by before a federal judge got around to ultimately deciding whether the case should revert back to state court. Until then, the state court had no jurisdiction and the case was in limbo. That was one of the primary reasons why defendants—especially well-heeled corporations hoping to grind down personal-injury victims—preferred that venue to state court.

This couldn't stand. Bill went to see Mark Griffin, who wasn't particularly worried. Jack in the Box's move was right out of the corporate defendant playbook, and Griffin had seen it before. The way around this, he insisted, was to simply file another class-action suit in another state court. Keller Rohrback just needed a new plaintiff, someone whose name didn't appear on the original class-action complaint. Thanks largely to Bill's media interviews, the firm had plenty of clients to choose from. Griffin agreed to draft a new complaint that could be filed in state court in Seattle.

The aggressive move was sure to send a clear signal to the Seattle legal community that Keller Rohrback was staking out its territory in the Jack in the Box litigation, but there was one problem. The Seattle legal community viewed Keller Rohrback primarily as an insurance-defense firm, not a plaintiffs' firm. And lawyers could be pretty territorial. In particular, tort lawyers didn't take kindly to having insurance lawyers trespass on their turf. There were already rumblings that Keller Rohrback was ill qualified to be leading the charge on behalf of injured children when the firm specialized in representing insurance companies, the likes of which would be doing Jack in the Box's bidding in a dispute like this.

A lot of this was petty bickering within the legal community. Nonetheless, it would be better for Keller Rohrback if these kinds of complaints didn't reach the court. At some point a judge would have to choose between the various class-action suits and the law firms that filed them. Only one complaint could be certified and only one firm would be named as the lead firm. Qualifications, expertise, and experience would matter in the selection process.

All of this was weighing on Bill's mind when he spent part of a weekend in February helping a fellow lawyer move from Seattle to Bainbridge Island. Shortly after he had been hired by Keller Rohrback, Bill had been introduced to Chris Pence, a lawyer who had attended law school with one of the senior partners at Bill's firm. Pence had opened a boutique personal-injury firm in Seattle called Pence & Dawson. Bill had remained a social acquaintance of Pence's and when he learned that Pence was relocating his family to Bainbridge Island, Bill volunteered his truck and his time.

Other than being lawyers and young fathers with a mutual friend, Bill and Pence had little in common. But that didn't stop Bill from helping Pence load his belongings onto the back of Bill's truck. They were busy talking about what lawyers talk about—their cases. Bill was going on about Jack in the Box when Pence mentioned that he had a client whose child had gotten sick in the outbreak.

"Hey Chris, I've got a brilliant idea."

"What?"

"You should join up with us," Bill said.

They were at a gas station filling up Bill's truck when this came up. Pence was intrigued. His firm was very small—just himself, one other partner, and an associate. Their practice was almost exclusively personal-injury work. They had zero experience with class-action suits or complex litigation. But they had a good reputation with the plaintiff's bar, and the opportunity to join forces with a big firm on the premier case in Seattle sounded promising.

Bill figured it could be the perfect marriage. Pence & Dawson was an answer to the claim that Keller Rohrback wasn't sufficiently established in the personal-injury world. And Keller Rohrback offered Pence & Dawson a chance to jump to the front of the line in litigating the case that every tort lawyer in Seattle wanted in on. When Bill put the idea to his partners, they embraced it and recommended the idea to Sarko, who saw no reason not to combine resources while gearing up to take on Jack in the Box. The partners, without Bill, brought Pence in for a meeting, and both sides agreed that the two firms would work as a team and share the fees.

Wednesday, February 24, 1993

With Suzanne looking on, Mike Canaan pressed his eye to the viewfinder on his camera and zoomed in on Brianne's body. Snapping shots, he worked his way down the large incision that ran down her torso. Before he'd seen Brianne, he'd never laid eyes on the internal organs of a living person. Without the lens creating some separation between him and Brianne's injuries, Canaan was sure he'd be unable to face what he was seeing. The damage was just too graphic. But that was precisely why these images needed to be captured. Jack in the Box and the meat industry needed to see why food safety had to become a higher priority.

Suddenly a priest entered the room to administer the last rites to Brianne. Respectfully, Canaan stepped away from the bed and bowed his head. After a few minutes, Canaan was able to finish photographing Brianne. Then he left Suzanne alone to contemplate the toughest decision of her life: whether to sign the papers authorizing the hospital to withdraw her daughter from life support.

Suzanne wasn't always sure that she believed in God. But she had convinced herself that God had finally spoken. And he was telling her that it was time to let Brianne go. Suzanne had done all a mother could do.

Before signing the authorization form, Suzanne needed someone to lean on, so, accompanied by her eldest daughter, Suzanne went to the pay phone down the hall from the ICU, where she placed a call to her pastor for spiritual guidance and support. While she was talking, she heard her name on the hospital's public address system: "Suzanne Kiner. Suzanne Kiner. Please come to the front desk."

"I'm being paged," Suzanne told her pastor in frustration. "Hold on."

Suzanne put her hand over the phone and turned to her teenage daughter. "Go find out what they want."

The daughter returned moments later. "They won't tell me. They want to talk to you. Now!"

That wasn't the answer Suzanne wanted to hear. "I have to go," she impatiently told her pastor before hanging up.

Just as Suzanne began to step away from the phone, the double swinging doors at the other end of the hallway flew open and two doctors ran toward her.

"She's awoken!" one of them shouted. "She's awoken!"

Suzanne Kiner was at Brianne's side moments after
her remarkable emergence from a coma.

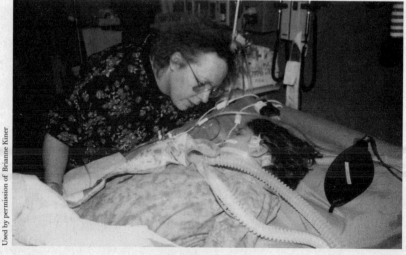

Steadied by two nurses, one on each arm, Suzanne entered Brianne's room. Brianne shifted her little brown eyes around the room, unable to move her head from side to side. It was clear she no idea where she was or how she had gotten there. She didn't know she was hooked up to a ventilator. She didn't know anything. She was just looking around like a newborn babe.

If she looks at me and knows who I am we'll be okay, Suzanne thought.

Suddenly Brianne's eyes met her mother's eyes and there was recognition.

"Oh God!" Suzanne cried out, and wept.

Later that day, Brianne's doctors warned Suzanne that the possibility that Brianne would die was still very real. No one knew how or if her body would hold up after sustaining such trauma to her vital organs. There was scant precedent in the medical literature of a person coming out of a prolonged coma after succumbing to HUS brought on by *E. coli* poisoning. The doctors wouldn't admit it, but they didn't know what to make of Brianne. In the absence of a medical explanation, only one word came to mind: *miracle.*

But everyone agreed that the next seven days would tell a lot. If Brianne made it through the week, her chances of recovery would be greatly improved. Until then, the hospital advised against making any public announcement about her emergence from a coma. With all the press her case had already attracted, word of her awakening was sure to touch off frenzy.

The change in Brianne's condition brought about a change in Suzanne, too. Suddenly she began thinking about all the things she'd neglected over the past forty days: medical bills, insurance forms, and domestic responsibilities. Plus there were all the new responsibilities she was about to face, extensive rehabilitation and medical care for her daughter being top on that list. Where to begin?

She called her older brother, Garry, in San Francisco with a simple plea: "Get me a lawyer."

Hubert agreed that the time had come to hire a Seattle lawyer. The case was about to take on a life of its own and there was only so much he could do from San Francisco. Assuming she survived, Brianne was going to need a staggering amount of medical care and rehabilitation. No doubt she'd have side effects from the illness that would stay with her throughout her life. Hubert wanted to insure that his sister got a top-flight personal-injury lawyer capable of handling such a complex case. He turned to Mike Canaan and gave him a simple charge: assemble a list of the top five trial lawyers in Seattle.

16

STRINGS ATTACHED

ON FEBRUARY 25 KELLER ROHRBACK FILED ITS SECOND CLASS-ACTION complaint: *Scott McKay v. Foodmaker, Inc.* This time the suit was brought in state court in Seattle, and Bill's phone started ringing as a result of the press coverage it drew. More parents wanted legal representation on behalf of their sick children. But one mother expressed fear that she might have forfeited her right to sue Jack in the Box. When Bill asked why, she said she had received a five-hundred-dollar check from the restaurant chain's insurance carrier. The words *FULL AND FINAL SETTLEMENT OF ALL CLAIMS* were printed on the check.

"Does this mean I can't sue them?" she asked.

First, Bill asked how she had come in contact with Jack in the Box's insurer.

The mother said she had seen a Jack in the Box advertisement in the newspaper. In it the company offered to pay all medical expenses. An 800 number was provided for parents to call.

Bill knew the ad well. He had a copy of it in his file. He asked what had happened when she called the 800 number.

The mother said an operator had taken her name and number. Later an insurance-claims adjuster had called and offered three hundred dollars for medical costs, plus two hundred dollars for pain and suffering. Figuring that was the best she could do, the mother had agreed.

"That's just bullshit," Bill said, assuring her that by cashing the check she was not foreclosing her right to sue the company.

Before long, Bill had a handful of clients who described a similar scenario. Then he found out that Chris Pence also had a client with one of these settlement checks. None of the checks exceeded a thousand dollars, and all of them contained the full-and-final-settlement language.

Bill and Pence huddled with Mark Griffin. "These greedy bastards think they can get away with this shit," Bill said, fuming.

"It's outrageous!" Pence thundered, insisting the practice was underhanded.

Griffin had seen corporations play hardball before, but he'd never had a case where virtually all of the victims were young children. Getting their parents to sign away their legal rights by tossing them a couple hundred bucks seemed over the top.

Attorney Mark Griffin played a key role in devising the strategy to bring a class-action suit against Jack in the Box.

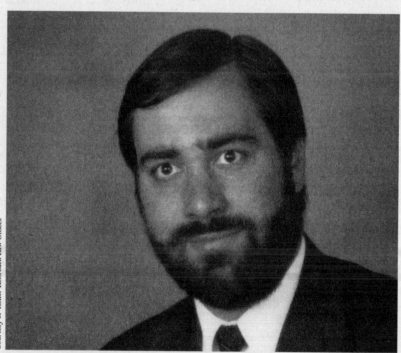

They all agreed something had to be done to challenge these settlement payoffs. But what?

Under Washington law, the injury claim of a minor couldn't be released simply by the act of a parent endorsing a check. Settlements involving minors had to be approved by a court. And before that could happen, a court-appointed guardian had to be named and the child had to be made aware of his or her legal rights and remedies.

But parents weren't familiar with these legal steps. And Jack in the Box's clever advertisement was enabling the company to sweep away claims by putting parents in direct contact with the insurance carrier. It irked Bill that the company was getting away with this by running an advertisement that promised to compensate parents with "no strings attached."

"Well, this," Bill said, waving one of his clients' settlement checks, "has strings attached."

Bill wanted to try to get a judge to issue an injunction to stop Jack in the Box. That got Griffin thinking. Since they had just filed a new class-action complaint, every child made sick by Jack in the Box meat was a potential class member. Under the federal rules of civil procedure, Jack in the Box was allowed to communicate with potential class members for the purposes of settlement. But Keller Rohrback's new suit had been filed in King County Superior Court in Seattle. And Griffin knew that King County had a unique exception to the federal rules, known as Local Rule 23, which prohibited defendants in a class-action suit from all contact with class members once a case was filed in a Seattle court. On the basis of Local Rule 23, Keller Rohrback could ask a Seattle judge to slap a temporary restraining order (TRO) on Jack in the Box.

Everyone agreed this was the best approach.

Yet none of them could point to a single example where a judge had ordered a company or its insurer to stop settling insurance claims under Local Rule 23. On a practical level, courts were very reluctant to interfere when people chose to settle directly with an insurance company rather than file a lawsuit. It wasn't the court's role to inform people that they had legal rights and were free to hire an attorney. That was the job of lawyers.

Nonetheless, the rule was on the books, so it seemed worth a try. Griffin talked to Sarko to see if he'd approve the idea.

Sarko liked the idea a lot and he saw nothing to lose by going for a TRO. If they succeeded, that would be pretty earth-shattering news in the sense that such a TRO had never been achieved before. And with other law firms contemplating class-action suits against Jack in the Box, Keller Rohrback would seize the upper hand. All the action would be focused on the McKay case. On the other hand, if they failed to get a TRO they'd be no worse off.

The more he thought about it, the more Sarko thought the court might just grant the TRO. "Add these things together," Sarko said. "A, an out-of-state corporation. B, children. C, harm. Is it really that hard, in this case, to get a judge to stay 'stop'?"

"We have to do this!" Griffin said, pounding his fist on Sarko's desk. "We have to stop these releases."

Sarko authorized Griffin to draft a motion and then take Marler along to argue for a TRO.

March 18, 1993

Suzanne Kiner wasn't used to press coverage. But she was getting used to the attention her daughter was commanding. It had been a week since Brianne had emerged from her coma. Not by choice, she had become an accidental celebrity, a miracle born of tragedy. After so many child illnesses and numerous deaths, the hospital felt it was appropriate to invite the media to meet Brianne and hear about her remarkable recovery. The city needed some good news.

Dr. John Neff, the medical director at Children's, led the news conference. "We didn't think she was going to make it at various times," Neff said. "To say this is a pleasant surprise is an understatement."

He provided an update on her condition. She was showing some signs of neurological recovery, although it was too early to say what her long-term progress would be on that front. But she was responding to simple questions from her parents and hospital staff by moving her head up and down for yes and side to side for no. She'd be remaining in the hospital for the foreseeable future before beginning a long period of physical therapy.

Reporters wanted to know what Brianne's future held.

"We can't tell if she will plateau at this level, or continue to improve, or if she continues to improve, how much she will improve," Neff said. "Right now, we're not ruling out any possibility. We hope for the absolute best."

Suzanne just beamed. She had her daughter back. She was alive! Nothing else mattered. She was alive!

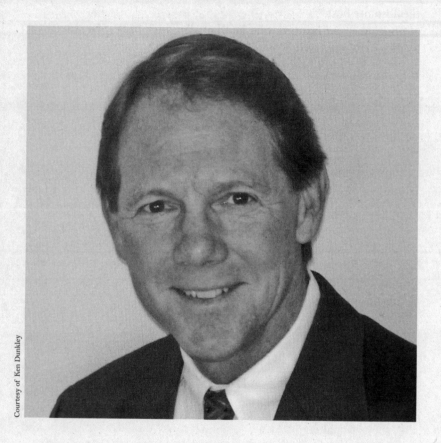

Ken Dunkley was blamed for not notifying his superiors at Jack in the Box that Washington State had raised the internal cooking temperature in hamburger to 155 degrees.

17

NOBODY BLAMES YOU

FRED GORDON'S HUNCH WAS ACCURATE. THE COMPANY *HAD* BEEN notified of the new cooking-temperature procedures in Washington. An internal audit of company records turned up a notice sent in May 1992 by one of the county health departments in Washington to corporate headquarters in San Diego. It detailed the more stringent cooking rules for beef. A second county in Washington had sent the same notice. The company had at least two documents in its files that indicated it was on notice of the rule change.

When faced with this information, Ken Dunkley was horrified. He suddenly recalled a staff meeting where someone had brought up this notice. It was in the summer of 1992.

"Someone mentioned that this document came from Washington State," explained Dunkley. "And there was something in it about cooking hamburger. We had a discussion around the table. We said that the national standard was 140 degrees. We talked about how we managed that. I don't remember what else happened."

The only other thing that Dunkley recalled about the staff meeting discussion pertaining to this notification was that everyone was more focused on the aspect of the document that dealt with chicken and *Salmonella*. The beef aspect of the notice was brushed over. In hindsight, this was a grave mistake.

Nugent wanted Dunkley fired. "He wasn't paying attention. He's the guy that really, really dropped the ball on this thing."

Gordon didn't think that was a wise idea. The discovery of the notices was embarrassing to Nugent personally and damaging to the company. But cutting Dunkley might make matters worse. The company was facing lawsuits on multiple fronts. It couldn't afford the risk of having a fired employee on the loose. Better to keep Dunkley in the fold.

Nugent didn't like it. It felt like the company had been failed by the quality-assurance team. Something like a rule change associated with a food poison risk was too damn dangerous to have been taken so lightly.

The decision on what to do about Dunkley was postponed. It would wait until after the annual shareholder meetings.

———————

Ken Dunkley didn't know where he stood. "I had questions in my mind about how I was viewed by the company," he explained. "I felt I was responsible, regardless of what the company position was. Not only was I not getting much sleep, but having to deal with the emotional aspect of it."

In the first week of March, Dunkley was sitting at his desk when a colleague entered his office. "Have you seen this?" said the colleague, dropping a newspaper on his desk. It was folded. The headline above the fold read: "Jack in the Box admits temperature rule error."

"You are named in the story," the colleague told him.

Anxiety swept over Dunkley as he started reading.

The article reported on comments made by Bob Nugent at the company's annual shareholder meeting. The report said that Nugent had told shareholders he had erred in his previous public statements that Jack in the Box had not known about the 155-degree meat-temperature regulation in Washington. On the contrary, Nugent told shareholders, he had since learned that in fact the company had been notified by health officials in Washington of the cooking-temperature increase. At least two official notices had turned up in Jack in the Box files. But those had never been shared with senior management.

Then Dunkley read the words that confirmed the guilt he'd been harboring.

> Nugent said the company's vice president of technical services is responsible for alerting senior management to such changes, but he had not done so with the Washington bulletin. Explaining that a board of directors committee is investigating why the two notices were ignored, Nugent said the company had "not yet decided what disciplinary action" to take.
>
> Ken Dunkley, the company's vice president of technical services, later was unavailable for comment.

Dunkley melted. Now he knew how the company viewed him—as a culprit. Seeing his name in print was like being forced to wear a scarlet letter. It was clear from the expression on his face that he needed a moment. His colleague stepped out and shut the door, leaving Dunkley alone.

Wounded, Dunkley read the article again. Tears streamed down his face. Everyone, he feared, would conclude that it was his fault that Jack in the Box had served undercooked meat that had killed children. He'd never felt more fallible, more desperate, more alone. Scared to leave his office, he reached for the phone and called his wife. He immediately told her about the article. "It names me as the person responsible," he said, weeping.

For almost two months Ken Dunkley had held himself together, but his wife could tell he was now coming unhinged. She dropped everything and rushed to corporate headquarters to try to console him.

By that afternoon, Dunkley received word that Foodmaker CEO Jack Goodall wanted to see him in his office. Just walking down the hall to Goodall's office was an exercise in shame, but the CEO had a firm message to deliver.

"You've done a lot for this company that's been really, really good," Goodall told him. "Nobody blames you."

Dunkley wanted to believe it. The trouble was that he blamed himself.

"You'll always have a place at Jack in the Box," Goodall assured him.

1
2
3
4
5
6
7

IN THE SUPERIOR COURT OF WASHINGTON FOR KING COUNTY

8 SCOTT McKAY, as guardian ad litem)
   of SARAH E. McKAY, a minor child,)   NO. 93-2-05171-9
9 individually and on behalf of   )
   themselves and all similarly   )   TEMPORARY RESTRAINING
10 situated,   )   ORDER AND ORDER SETTING
)   HEARING ON MOTION FOR
11   Plaintiffs,   )   PRELIMINARY INJUCTION
)
12   v.   )
)
13 FOODMAKER, INC., a Delaware   )
   corporation doing business as   )
14 "JACK-IN-THE-BOX" RESTAURANTS,   )
)
15   Defendant.   )
)
16 _____)

17   THIS MATTER having come before the Court in the above-
18 captioned matter on a motion of Plaintiffs Scott McKay,
19 individually and as guardian ad litem for his minor child, Sarah
20 E. McKay (age 4) for a Temporary Restraining Order enjoining
21 defendant Foodmaker, Inc., doing business as "Jack-In-The-Box"
22 Restaurants, and their employees, agents, independent contractors,
23 insurance companies, and all others acting in concert with them
24 from contacting, speaking with or attempting to obtain in any
25 manner whatsoever any release or settlement of claims in any way
26 relating to the contamination of food products from any individual

to obtain in any manner what-
claims in any way relating to
om any individual unless such
urt. Nothing in this order
he medical expenses of such
f such medical expenses are
release or settlement.

dant shall appear before the
lendar on the _16_ day of
o'clock _A_.m. to show cause
t be entered continuing this
action.

iffs shall post cash/bond in
Clerk of this Court pursuant
of this injunction. Unless
Temporary Restraining Order

_1993_

ay of _March_

Superior Court Commissioner

TEMPORARY RESTRAINING ORDER - 3
H:\CLIENTS\20983\1\TRO1.ORD

KELLER ROHRBACK
SUITE 3200
1201 THIRD AVENUE
SEATTLE, WASHINGTON 98101-3052
(206) 623-1900

A pivotal moment in the litigation came when a Seattle judge issued this restraining order against Jack in the Box.

18

A SHITLOAD OF MONEY

Wednesday, March 3, 1993
Karr Tuttle Campbell Law Office
Seattle, Washington

IT WAS IMPOSSIBLE NOT TO STARE AT HER. SEATED ON A BED WITH her legs partially tucked under her, she wore nothing but a silky, see-through top that was wide open, exposing her large, voluptuous breasts. The tips of her nipples were barely obscured by a pink strand of fabric. The negligee was tied closed at her waist with a sash.

The three-foot high original oil painting didn't exactly fit the office decor of Seattle law firm Karr Tuttle Campbell. The portrait was a bit too racy—not to mention downright tacky—for a firm whose clients included some of the leading banks, corporations, and insurance firms on the West Coast. But none of that fazed attorney Bob Piper, a longtime partner who had mounted the painting right above the wooden credenza in his twenty-sixth-story corner office. With a pot belly and a bulbous nose, Piper resembled a penguin when he walked, and he tended to sweat profusely, even when sitting still. He swore like a sailor and drank like one, too. When introducing himself to new associates at the firm, he'd say: "I'm really good at two things, trying cases and screwing women."

Seated beneath his infamous nude painting, Piper marveled at the morning paper's headline—"*E. Coli* Victim Out of Coma." He couldn't get over the fact that Brianne Kiner had come back after forty days in a coma. He'd been tracking the *E. coli* outbreak from the moment public-health officials pinned it on Jack in the Box. Having spent decades representing companies facing big liability exposure, Piper knew very early on that many aspects of the *Jack in the Box* case would come down to insurance—hundreds of sick children meant hundreds of claims.

More than any other, Brianne Kiner's situation captivated Piper. If she had died as everyone had expected, the insurance company would have gotten off easy. In insurance terms, the worth of a deceased child is about two hundred thousand dollars. But when Brianne Kiner woke up, Jack in the Box's exposure went into orbit. Of the hundreds of injured children in the outbreak, none had sustained injuries as severe as Brianne's. Doctors were sure she'd die from all the organ damage. Her odds-defying survival would surely mean years of rehabilitation, organ transplants, surgeries, and medications that would all add up to big, big money. Jack in the Box—which is to say, its insurers—would be on the hook to pay all of it.

"This is going to be the biggest case ever," Piper told a colleague. "And this kid is the poster child for the biggest case ever. It's an unbelievable case!"

Meanwhile, the media couldn't get enough of Brianne's inspiring twist to an otherwise tragic story. The situation was a chamber of horrors for Jack in the Box. Personal-injury lawyers were already jockeying to represent Brianne Kiner in a lawsuit that had sky-is-the-limit potential for damage claims.

But what Piper wanted was to defend Jack in the Box. The restaurant chain's nightmare was his opportunity. If he could get control of the defense, he'd have a mighty long stream of lucrative, high-profile defense work. His problem was that Jack in the Box already had a law firm handling the insurance claims. Seattle's Lee, Smart, Cook, Martin & Patterson had been chosen by Jack in the Box's insurer CNA. And David Martin, a partner at the firm, took the lead. It's standard practice for restaurant chains to have a primary insurer that is responsible for covering the kind of day-to-day claims that emerge in the restaurant business—slip-and-falls and other things of that nature. CNA held a $1 million policy for such claims.

But the primary insurer is only the first layer of insurance. Restaurant chains will purchase additional insurance—known as excess layers—to cover larger catastrophic claims. Chubb had the next layer—a $10 million policy. As soon as the CNA money ran out, Chubb would step in as the primary insurer.

Piper had done a lot of work for Chubb over the years and maintained a very close relationship with their adjusters. Piper placed a call his best contact at Chubb and discussed the Jack in the Box situation. He learned that there was a lot more insurance money behind Chubb's.

Most fast-food restaurant chains held anywhere between $20 million and $40 million worth of excess liability insurance. But less than a year before the outbreak, Jack in the Box had added Paul Carter to its board of directors. He'd been a longtime insurance consultant. The first thing he did was analyze Jack in the Box's insurance coverage and determine the company was dangerously underinsured. Acting on Carter's recommendation, the company upped its liability coverage to $100 million. If Jack in the Box survived the outbreak, Piper believed the decision to increase its insurance would be the primary reason why. He had the breakdown of the carriers and the amount of their policies:

- Chubb: $10 million.
- Transamerica: $20 million.
- AIG: $5 million.
- Home: $40 million.
- Chubb: $15 million.
- Fireman's Fund: $15 million.

By the time Piper hung up with Chubb, he was rubbing his hands together. *One hundred million dollars is a shitload of money*, he kept telling himself. He had an idea for how to wrest control of Jack in the Box's defense. But first he needed to make sure his idea was legal. That would require some legal research, which was something Piper didn't do. That was what associates were for. He went looking for the firm's newest junior associate.

At 5'6" and 140 pounds, thirty-two-year-old Denis Stearns would have been easily mistaken for a college student interning at Karr Tuttle

Campbell. His glasses with giant round lenses sandwiched between smooth boyish cheeks and thick wavy brown hair didn't help matters. When Stearns smiled you expected to see braces.

Fresh out of law school at the University of Wisconsin, Stearns made sure to at least dress maturely: black, lace-up wing tip shoes, a white shirt, and a Brooks Brothers, classic, two-button, navy blue suit. His wardrobe never varied. Neither did his work habits. Every day he showed up early and stayed late. Karr Tuttle Campbell liked those qualities in its associates.

Stearns had something else going for him, an unusual knack for performing fast, extensive legal research. Partners like an associate who knows his way around the law library. Digging through case law and cross-referencing with the most recent court opinions is the blue-collar side of a white-collar world. Here's where Stearns had a leg up. He came from a blue-collar family. His father drove a dump truck and he had a stay-at-home mom. No one else in his family had attended college. Therefore, education had not been a high priority in the home he grew up in outside Seattle.

But Stearns was intellectually oriented and turned out to be smarter than most of the smart kids. The trouble was he had no friends. An outsider, he ended up spending a lot of time in the library, which turned him into a voracious reader and introduced him to the best of friends—books. Stories by Ernest Hemmingway and F. Scott Fitzgerald were among his favorites. But nothing grabbed him like *A Portrait of the Artist as a Young Man* by James Joyce. He read it multiple times. It was easy to memorize the passage that seemed like it had been written just for him.

> Mother is putting my new secondhand clothes in order. She prays now, she says, that I may learn in my own life and away from home and friends what the heart is and what it feels. Amen. So be it. Welcome, O life! I go to encounter for the millionth time the reality of experience and to forge in the smithy of my soul the uncreated conscience of my race.

It was after reading this that Stearns dropped out of high school before the conclusion of his senior year and left home. Desperate for separation, he went all the way to LA. He floundered at first, before landing a retail sales job and completing his GED. But what really got his life on track was coming to terms with the fact that he was gay—and that it was okay. In high school he'd privately experienced infatuations with male friends. But now he was free to let his heart feel.

Self-assured, he headed back to Seattle and ended up at Seattle University majoring in philosophy, which got him interested in legal theory. To pay the bills he took a job as an office assistant at Keller Rohrback. By then he was contemplating law school and he figured he might as well find out what it was like to practice law. He sorted the mail, delivered faxes, accepted deliveries, set up conference rooms, and ultimately became responsible for opening the office on Saturdays, which included bringing the donuts.

Naturally, Stearns crossed paths often with the secretary to the firm's managing partner Lynn Sarko. Sarko's secretary was a single mother who always seemed to have some man drama going on in her life. Stearns became a great sounding board for her. There was something about being gay that gave Stearns an ability to hit it off with women having man problems. Stearns's relationship with Sarko's secretary opened the door for access to Sarko. And at some point, Stearns put it out there that he was contemplating law school.

Sarko took a liking to Stearns and lobbied him to apply to law school at the University of Wisconsin, where he had been editor of the law review. Sarko even wrote a letter of recommendation on Stearns's behalf. Stearns excelled at Wisconsin and upon graduation ended up getting hired by Karr Tuttle Campbell, one of Keller Rohrback's competitors. The two firms were located in the same office tower and were separated by just a few floors. That was when Stearns first crossed paths with Bob Piper.

To Piper, being gay was as understandable as being from Mars. But he saw in Stearns the same qualities that Sarko had seen: brains, attention to detail, reliability, and a great work ethic. And with the scheme that Piper had in mind, Stearns was just the man for the job.

Saying nothing, Piper motioned for Stearns to follow him.

Stearns grabbed a yellow legal pad and a pen and hustled down to Piper's office.

"Close the door," Piper said.

Stearns took a seat.

"Have you seen what's going on with Jack in the Box?" Piper asked.

Stearns nodded. Like everyone else, he'd been following the story in the media. He'd also been talking to other lawyers about the case.

"There will be a shitload of lawsuits," Piper said. "A shitload."

Stearns raised his eyebrows and nodded in agreement.

"Look, I'm going to make a play for that work," Piper said.

A play? Stearns didn't get it. Karr Tuttle Campbell was an insurance-defense firm. It was common knowledge that Jack in the Box and its insurer CNA had already chosen Lee, Smart, Cook, Martin & Patterson as its defense firm and that David Martin was handling the case.

Piper explained that Jack in the Box would run through the $1 million policy with CNA in no time. The next insurer was Chubb, and Piper had been doing work for Chubb for years.

Hmm. Stearns was starting to get the picture, sort of.

"I have a research project I need you to do right away," said Piper. He laid out two tasks:

- First, find out what legal basis existed for Jack in the Box to dismiss David Martin's firm.

- Second, look into whether Piper's past work for Chubb would preclude him from representing Jack in the Box. In other words, was there a conflict of interest that would prevent Chubb's former lawyer from becoming Jack in the Box's new one?

Eager to get started, Stearns got up and headed for the door.

But Piper stopped him with one more instruction: "Be sure not to write anything down," he advised Stearns. "Just come back and report to me."

Only a few months removed from law school, Stearns's ethical antenna went up.

Piper sensed Stearns was uneasy, but figured Stearns would get over it. Meantime, Piper wanted no evidence that he had advised Chubb on the legal steps for getting Jack in the Box to dump Martin and hire him. "We can't be seen as giving advice to the insurance company if we're defending someone they insure," Piper said.

"Got it," Stearns said, promising to have answers to Piper's legal questions as quickly as possible.

Four floors above Piper's office, Bill Marler and Mark Griffin put the finishing touches on a motion asking the court to stop Jack in the Box and its insurance companies from settling with *E. coli* victims. They scanned the wording one more time:

> THIS MATTER having come before the Court on a motion of Plaintiffs Scott McKay, individually and as guardian ad litem for his minor child, Sarah E. McKay (age 4) for a Temporary Restraining Order enjoining defendant Foodmaker, Inc., doing business as "Jack-In-The-Box" Restaurants, and their employees, agents, independent contractors, insurance companies, and all others acting in concert with them from contacting, speaking with or attempting to obtain in any manner whatsoever any release or settlement of claims in any way relating to the contamination of food products from any individual unless the content of such communications are approved by the Court.

Along with the Motion, Griffin attached an order for a judge to sign. He included some critical language in the order: "Nothing in this order prevents defendant from paying for the medical expenses of such individuals so long as the payment of such medical expenses are not conditional upon the signing of a release or settlement."

Bill faxed copies to Chris Pence to review. Then he dispatched a courier to hand-deliver the paperwork to David Martin's office before hustling off to the courthouse with Griffin. While waiting in line to see the judge assigned to hear civil motions, Bill kept looking over his shoulder, expecting to see Martin come bursting into the room at any moment to contest the request for a TRO. But by the time Griffin handed the papers up to the judge, Martin hadn't shown.

After reading the papers over, the judge handed them back. He wanted nothing to do with the matter and instructed them to go see the court's presiding judge.

Bill had known this was going to be controversial, but he hadn't expected the motions judge to pass the petition off like a hot potato. Neither had Griffin.

They headed upstairs, where they were told the presiding judge would be unavailable until after lunch. It was after 1:30 by the time the presiding judge returned to the bench. He looked over the papers. But before hearing anything from Griffin or Bill, he had one question: "Where's your opposing counsel?"

Griffin said they didn't know.

The judge asked if the other side had been properly notified.

Bill confirmed that at 10:54 a.m. the law firm of David Martin had received notice of Keller Rohrback's intention to seek the restraining order.

The judge looked at the clock. Just over three hours had gone by. Technically, Griffin and Bill had met their obligation to notify— but just barely. The judge preferred Martin be present and have an opportunity to contest the motion. Ex parte proceedings were frowned on. He instructed the two attorneys to call Martin and find out whether he intended to show.

Bill and Griffin stepped outside. Neither was eager to talk to Martin. Griffin placed the call, and a receptionist indicated she wasn't sure of Martin's whereabouts. She put Griffin through to Martin's direct line, which went to an answering machine.

Thank God.

Griffin left a very brief message.

Still not satisfied, the presiding judge instructed his clerk to try reaching Martin. Anxious, Bill kept looking at his watch, convinced that Martin would enter the courtroom at any moment.

After a while the clerk reported that he had had no luck reaching Martin either.

The judge called Bill and Griffin forward. He'd studied the motion. It wasn't clear why he should order Jack in the Box to stop obtaining settlements from people who wanted to settle.

Bill had a copy of a two-hundred-dollar settlement check from the mother of an ill child. Bill contrasted this with what Jack in the Box had said to the media: On January 22, 1993, Jack in the Box's president, Robert Nugent, had told the *Seattle Post-Intelligencer*: "We intend to do what is right by the people affected. We will do what is morally right. We are not going to sit down and negotiate with people." The next day Jack in the Box's parent company, Foodmaker, Inc., established its 800 number to answer questions about the *E. coli* outbreak. Then on February 1, Nugent publicly announced that Jack in the Box would pay hospitalization costs of customers sickened by the *E. coli* bacterium, vowing to help the restaurant chain's customers "immediately, with no strings attached."

But there were strings attached to two-hundred-dollar settlement check. And speaking of two hundred dollars, there was nothing right or moral about it.

Griffin piled on, arguing that the 800 number was really being used to put sick people—for the most part children—in contact with Jack in the Box's insurance carrier in order to trick them into accepting settlement checks that precluded the recipients' right to bring suit against the restaurant chain down the road. That was contrary to the public pronouncements of Jack in the Box's president, Robert Nugent. More important, the parents calling the 800 number were at the disadvantage of being without legal representation while negotiating with a sophisticated insurance company.

The judge had heard enough. At 2:52 p.m. he signed the order, stopping Jack in the Box's insurers from settling with food poisoning victims without court approval. The TRO was set to expire on March 17. Both sides were ordered to reappear on March 16 to argue for and against making the injunction permanent.

Bill's heart began pounding. Griffin tried to remain stoic, but he realized they had just pulled off a major coup. Griffin couldn't wait to tell Sarko. Bill couldn't wait to call the press.

The Seattle media jumped on the TRO story and Jack in the Box came off like a duplicitous corporation putting profits ahead of injured customers.

The moment the news of the TRO hit the street, Martin was in court trying to get it dissolved. He had a series of complaints. "This lawsuit was served on my client on March 3," he told the court. "I didn't even know about the lawsuit when they came up and got a TRO. It was unknown to me."

Martin had an even bigger complaint about the language of the order itself. "This order," he told a judge, "was clearly inappropriate. . . . The language prohibited us . . . from contacting anybody and talking with anyone about settlement, whether they were represented or unrepresented." From Martin's point of view, the order went way too far.

After listening to Martin, the judge directed him and Keller Rohrback to try to negotiate a revised order that was agreeable to both sides. Until then, the existing order would remain in place.

Bob Nugent hit the roof when his VP over public relations informed him they were getting calls from reporters in Seattle wanting to know why Jack in the Box was trying to shortchange children who were hospitalized in the outbreak. Specifically, a Seattle lawyer—Bill Marler—had accused Nugent and the restaurant chain of telling the public one thing with its advertising campaign, while using its insurance company to do something entirely different. It irritated Nugent that some lawyer was taking potshots at him. He was even angrier that Jack in the Box's lawyer in Seattle had set him and the company up to look bad. Nugent had been unaware that Jack in the Box's insurer was settling insurance claims on the cheap. Fred Gordon hadn't known it either.

"How can we be saying we're going to take care of you and then screwing you?" Nugent said.

"It looks like you're trying to con people," Gordon said.

"How can anyone be so damn stupid?" Nugent said.

"Anybody who would do that has no brains," Gordon said.

"Why would we want someone like that representing us?" Nugent said. Gordon agreed.

19

PICKPOCKET

March 16, 1993

BILL MARLER WAS LOOKING FORWARD TO GOING BACK TO COURT TO argue against Martin over the merits of the TRO. But Sarko, had taken an increased interest in the case and chose to take the lead. Over the previous two weeks, Keller Rohrback and David Martin's office had failed to agree on language that would replace the TRO. The two sides were left with no choice but to bring their impasse to a judge. Sarko asked Griffin to handle the oral argument. Pence and Bill accompanied him.

"Well, Your Honor, we've exchanged drafts of the proposed notice, and it turns out that the parties are worlds apart," Griffin said. Then he reminded the judge of the dispute's short history. "Initially, this matter, a class-action case, was filed in Pierce County court by my law firm, and at the time we advised Mr. Martin and the other lawyers representing Jack in the Box of Local Rule 23 of this court, which prohibits all contact with class members once a class-action case is filed in this court."

Griffin explained that Jack in the Box had reacted to this by filing a motion to get the case transferred to federal court. "At the same time," Griffin continued, "Foodmaker filed an affidavit which indicated, in fact, Foodmaker was utilizing the 1-800 number not just to pay medical expenses of the victims of the *E. coli* outbreak, but also to seek releases of claims from class members, including the claims of minors without advising these people of their rights."

This got the judge's attention. He looked directly at Griffin. "You say they filed an affidavit to that effect?"

"No," Martin interjected.

"Yes they did, Your Honor," Griffin countered.

"No, we didn't, Your Honor," Martin insisted. "I signed an affidavit—"

"I'm going to hear from you in a moment," the judge said, cutting Martin off.

"I know," Martin continued. "But that's a falsehood."

"Well, you can tell me that when I get to you," the judge said.

Griffin couldn't even get through his opening statement without a testy exchange with Martin. He closed by defending his firm's decision to seek a TRO, insisting that Jack in the Box and its parent company, Foodmaker, were, in fact, seeking settlements with minors who did not have adequate notice of their legal rights. For that reason, he insisted, the court had to make the injunction permanent.

Martin told a very different story. "Your Honor, it's not really all that complicated. I'm David Martin, representing Foodmaker, Inc., and Jack in the Box. There's been some blatant misrepresentations presented to you today, and I don't mean to start out with that, but it's true."

After criticizing Keller Rohrback's tactics in securing the TRO, Martin immediately attacked the order. "The language prohibited us," he began, "from contacting anybody and talking with anyone about settlement, whether they were represented or unrepresented."

For Martin, Keller Rohrback had gotten way ahead of itself by seeking a TRO. The way he saw things, it wasn't even clear that the *E. coli* outbreak was worthy of a class-action lawsuit. "Bodily injury claims like this have never traditionally been held to be class-actions," he said. "Look at the asbestos litigation. They aren't class-actions. And the reason why is because the individual damage claim of each person is different."

Martin made it clear that he was prepared to challenge whether it was even appropriate for Keller Rohrback to pursue a class-action.

"Before they can start out sending notices like they're suggesting be sent, they have to have a class-action certified," he argued.

It was clear that all of these issues weren't going to be easily sorted out. The presiding judge assigned the dispute to another judge and scheduled oral arguments. He instructed both sides to prepare written summaries and have them on the judge's desk prior to the next court appearance.

Lawyers were trying to explain to Bob Nugent why the approach taken by David Martin made perfect legal sense. Not all of the children swept up in the outbreak had sustained life-threatening or serious injuries. Some experienced only diarrhea and stomach cramps and were treated and released after incurring only modest medical expenses. From a business standpoint, it made financial sense to try to extinguish those claims as quickly and economically as possible. That was pretty standard operating procedure in the insurance business.

Nugent slammed his fist down on the desk. "I don't give a shit!" he said, fuming. "These people shouldn't have to come crawling to us."

Nugent was tired of working so hard to save the company while lawyers insisted on approaches that were causing the company's image to take a beating in the press.

"I just want to do what's right, damn it," he continued. "And the right thing to do is own up to responsibility and pay for these poor people who had to put their kids in the hospital."

The latest dustup over the TRO was the last straw. He was ready to fire some lawyers—as soon as he could find a replacement for them.

His legal research complete, Denis Stearns rushed into Bob Piper's office with the results. As a general rule, insurance companies chose the law firm to represent the insured. So, in this case, CNA had selected David Martin's firm to defend Jack in the Box against claims by those who had gotten sick from eating bad meat. CNA was paying the claims and therefore had the prerogative to pick Jack in the Box's defense lawyer.

Yeah, yeah, yeah. Piper knew that much. What about changing firms?

Stearns was getting to that.

Once a law firm was selected by an insurer, the customary practice was for the firm to remain in place even though the insurance carriers might change. So once CNA's $1 million policy was used up and Chubb's $10 million policy kicked in, Martin would remain in place as the lawyer.

However, if Jack in the Box alleged an act of bad faith that further injured the restaurant chain, then the company could insist on new legal representation. Bad faith could consist of any strategy or conduct by the law firm or the insurance company that did harm to the insured.

Attorney Bob Piper, shown here holding two glasses of wine, convinced Jack in the Box to hire him to represent the company in the class-action suit filed by the parents of injured children.

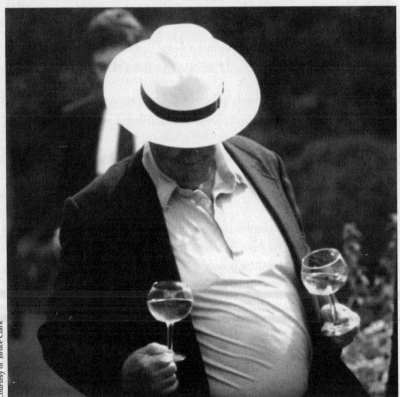

Courtesy of Bruce Clark

Piper let out a bellowing laugh and flung himself back in his chair, slamming his thick hands on the arm rests and letting his big gut bulge out. "This is great," he thundered, his face red with delight.

Stearns wasn't sure what was so great about what he'd just said.

Piper pointed to the headline in the *Seattle Times*: "Jack-In-Box Agrees to Quit Asking for Releases from *E. coli* Victims."

The bottom line was that after two days of oral arguments, a temporary agreement had been reached between Keller Rohrback and David Martin. Piper tossed the paper to Stearns, who began reading.

> The owner of the Jack in the Box fast-food chain has agreed to stop eliciting signed releases from *E. coli* poisoning victims when it negotiates to pay their medical bills.

> Under an agreement filed yesterday in King County Superior Court, Foodmaker, Inc., may continue using a toll-free telephone line to locate victims and arrange to pay medical bills. But the company agreed to stop asking victims to promise they will never sue for more money.

> The agreement nullifies a temporary restraining order issued this week.

> "The only thing we were worried about was the releases," said Lynn Sarko, one of the lawyers who sought the restraining order. "We've had people sign releases for as little as $200 or $300. If you got sick and were passing blood and everything, I would think the sheer fright of it would be worth more than $200."

> Releases already signed are viewed as binding by the company, said Wiley Brooks, a press spokesman for Jack in the Box.

Stearns handed the article back to Piper. Jack in the Box came off looking terrible.

That was why Piper liked it so much. The press was having a field day with the story at Jack in the Box's expense.

Stearns saw Piper's point. *But how does that help him become Jack in the Box's lawyer?* he wondered.

The idea of taking over the defense in a massive foodborne illness outbreak that was generating national headlines seemed like a pipe dream. But Stearns had learned not to doubt Piper, who had a brilliant mind for problem solving. More than anything, though, Piper was a master salesman. Juries were mesmerized by his courtroom performances. He was so effective that he had once seduced an attractive female juror to the point that she married him after he won the trial.

Piper was going to need all these skills to persuade Jack in the Box to give him control of the company's defense against Brianne Kiner and the hundreds of other victims in Seattle.

Stearns sat back in his chair as Piper picked up the phone and called Chubb. With the insurer's $10 million policy about to kick in, the time had come to arrange a face-to-face meeting between Piper and the top brass at Jack in the Box.

With Denis Stearns in tow, Bob Piper strolled through a series of long hallways that snaked through a warehouse-like building. Eventually they reached a conference room with a large wooden table surrounded by high-back leather chairs on wheels. Piper took the middle seat on one side. Stearns sat immediately to his left.

Nugent entered from another door, flanked by attorney Fred Gordon and Dave Theno and other members of the company's board of directors. The tension in the room was palpable. Stearns's stomach was in knots. Piper couldn't wait to get down to business.

A deft observer of public perception, Piper recognized that Jack in the Box was facing an image nightmare: dead kids, claims in various states, the CEO being hauled before Congress for a public tongue-lashing, and a press cycle that kept churning out nonstop stories about *E. coli* that always mentioned Jack in the Box.

With the company's leadership basically in the fetal position, Piper made things sound as perilous as possible. This dark tone made Stearns uneasy. *Why not give Jack in the Box a reason to be encouraged?*

Piper was getting to that. But first he wanted to get hired. And to do that he needed to scare them into believing he was the only one capable of bailing them out of the mess they were in. That led him to Dave Martin. Without mentioning Martin's name, Piper railed against the typical insurance-defense tactics. That style worked well in some types of litigation, but it was no way to respond in a case involving victims that were little children made deathly ill by your product. This was a time for diplomacy and negotiation, not a short fuse. The last thing Jack in the Box needed was a lawyer out in front with a bad temper.

Nugent nodded as Piper mercilessly threw Martin under the bus. For the first time in a long time Nugent felt like he was listening to a lawyer who spoke his language.

Piper continued. Instead of assuring Jack in the Box that its legal problems were manageable, he took the unorthodox approach of insisting the sky was falling, reminding them that there would be lawsuits in multiple states.

"You can't have lawyers in each state in charge," Piper said. "You need one firm in control. Every case should be run out of our office. Nothing gets filed in a court without my approval."

The meeting lasted for just over an hour. After fielding a few questions, Piper and Stearns left. Then Jack in the Box officials discussed what to do.

"I liked him," Gordon said. "He has a global vision."

Dave Theno agreed.

The other executives in the room were comfortable with Piper, too. Mostly, they were all so furious with David Martin's firm that they were ready to pull the trigger.

For Nugent it was an easy call. The way things had been handled up in Seattle had been disastrous for the company. Piper was a lawyer who spoke more like a businessman. He understood that the top priority was saving the company.

Nugent gave his instructions: fire Martin's firm and hire Piper's. And do it fast.

As soon as Piper and Stearns boarded the plane in San Diego to head back to Seattle, Piper plopped down in his first-class seat and asked the stewardess for some vodka. "Give me two bottles," he said.

Then he turned to Stearns. "You're only as good as your book of business," he said, laughing raucously.

Stearns knew what that meant. A lawyer is only as good as his list of clients. That's why Piper was feeling so good. By picking David Martin's pocket, Piper just added a big client to his book: Jack in the Box.

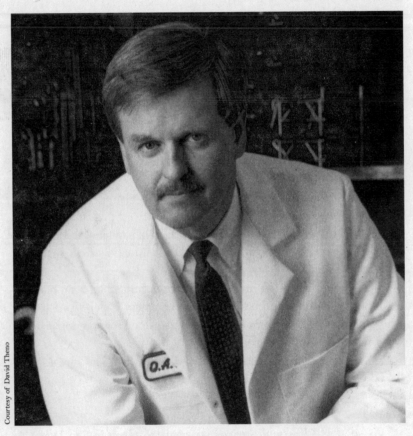

Dave Theno was put in charge of quality assurance
for Jack in the Box.

20

GEARING UP

Mike Canaan had connections to some of the top corporate lawyers in Seattle. But he didn't know any personal-injury lawyers. So he called a corporate lawyer he'd done work for and asked him to recommend the top five lawyers he'd choose to represent Brianne Kiner. Canaan ended up with a virtual who's who list of Seattle's top tort lawyers.

After reviewing the names, Garry Hubert instructed Canaan to contact each lawyer on the list and set up interviews with them. Hubert planned to fly up from San Francisco to vet the various lawyers to determine which one was best suited to represent Brianne's interests.

Bob Piper liked minions and Denis Stearns didn't mind being one. The role provided him a chance to work hand-in-hand with a senior partner on a case that dominated the headlines. Although it would be a couple of weeks before the transition was complete and Piper officially took control of the case from David Martin's office, there was a lot to do to get ready.

"We're going to need more people on this case," Piper told Stearns. "Who do you think we should get?"

Stearns didn't feel qualified to recommend someone. He hadn't been at the firm long enough.

Piper asked Stearns how he felt about Bruce Clark, a thirty-seven-year-old junior partner who had joined the firm right out of law school.

Besides Piper, Clark was one of the few lawyers Stearns had worked with. They were doing a maritime case together. Stearns couldn't have enough good things to say about him.

Piper put Clark on the team. Clark had an unusually soft touch for a lawyer. Nobody at the firm spoke quite like him. He would have made a great diplomat. That was why Piper wanted him.

As soon as Clark sat down beside Stearns, Piper looked across his desk and brought him up to speed on the case. Then he talked about roles.

Stearns would handle all legal research and oversee the discovery process. Soon plaintiffs' lawyers would be seeking all sorts of documents from Jack in the Box in an attempt to show negligence. Piper wanted Stearns to learn every aspect of Jack in the Box's operations and quality assurance, backward and forward.

Clark would handle all court appearances and be responsible for interfacing with insurance adjusters and medical experts. Jack in the Box needed a more conciliatory advocate in the courtroom and someone astute enough to understand some pretty complicated medicine and science.

Piper planned to be the general. He would communicate directly with the higher-ups at Jack in the Box, the insurance companies and the opposing law firms. Nothing was to happen without his approval.

When the meeting broke up, Clark and Stearns compared notes. Clark was thrilled to join the team. He'd worked with Piper on some smaller cases in the past. So he knew all about his eccentricities and volatile temper. But he really liked Piper.

"How could you not like a guy with the balls to have a cheesy portrait of a nude woman on his office wall?" Clark said.

Stearns laughed.

For Dave Theno, decision day had come: remain a consultant or sell his business and become an employee at Jack in the Box.

On paper the decision looked pretty clear. Theno & Associates was a lucrative consulting firm with healthy revenue projections for the foreseeable future. As his own boss, Theno was taking home close to a quarter of a million dollars a year in personal income. Conversely, Jack in the Box was a big corporation in big trouble. Bankruptcy loomed if something remarkable didn't happen to reverse the impact of the outbreak. Leaving a thriving business for one on the brink of failure just didn't make sense.

But Theno couldn't overlook one thing. Over his twenty-five-year career in the food industry, he'd never gotten to make his mark. He'd worked with restaurants, ranchers, and large-scale food-processing companies. He'd worked with government regulators and sat on high-level advisory committees. But in all those instances his mandate was to tweak the system, not revolutionize it. Jack in the Box was offering him a chance to try to do something that no one thought could be done—come up with a state-of-the-art food-safety-hazard plan for fresh meat. It was the kind of radical approach that a national fast-food chain would never consider under normal circumstances. But the *E. coli* outbreak had changed all that. It was an opportunity, Theno realized, that might not come again.

He told his partners which way he was leaning. Then he went to see Nugent.

"Bob, if I do this I'm going to need a tremendous amount of support from you," he said.

Nugent promised that he'd have it.

Theno wanted two more things out of Nugent. The first was a heart-to-heart conversation about personal beliefs and values. Nugent agreed and for the next two hours the two men talked about their parents, their upbringing, their wives, and their priorities in life. Satisfied, Theno turned to his final request—an assurance that whatever he designed would be shared with the industry.

"Absolutely," Nugent told him. "If McDonald's had shared, even on a private basis with the industry, maybe this could have been precluded."

The only thing left to discuss was money. Nugent asked how much Theno expected to make.

"Bob, I'm giving up a good business," he said. "To some extent I'm taking a gamble. I just want you guys to be fair."

Nugent promised to match his annual salary as a consultant, plus provide benefits and options that were not available as a consultant. The two men shook hands.

"Let's get to work, partner," Theno said.

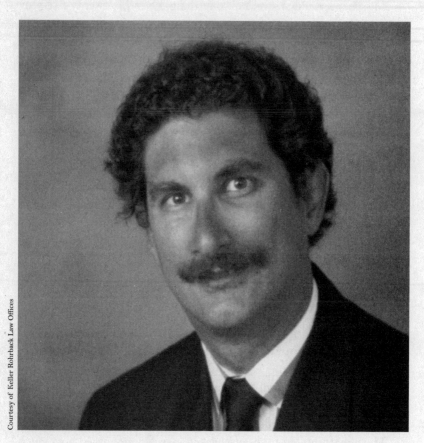

Lynn Sarko was the managing partner at Keller Rohrback when the firm brought a massive class-action suit against Jack in the Box.

21

THE DEVIL YOU KNOW

JACK IN THE BOX'S LAWYER, DAVID MARTIN, HAD BEEN CHALLENGING Keller Rohrback's attempt to establish a class of plaintiffs to sue the restaurant chain. But when he took over, Bob Piper had no intention of challenging the certification of the class-action. He wanted to settle the claims against Jack in the Box, not contest them. He planned to treat the class-action suit as a device to extinguish hundreds of cases without having to litigate them individually.

There was another advantage to a class-action approach. Rather than deal with scores of lawyers, Piper could deal largely with one firm on all the less severe cases. That would make the claims much more manageable and allow Piper to focus more attention on the larger individual cases, such as Kiner.

Like water, Piper gravitated toward the path of least resistance. That meant identifying one law firm that would be easy to work with. A number of firms had filed class-action suits, but ultimately, only one class would be certified and one firm would be selected to represent the class. Technically, Piper had no say in which firm got chosen. But since he would be the one handing out Jack in the Box's money, he planned to use the power of the purse to help insure that he'd be dealing with a firm that would be most receptive to speedy settlements. In his mind, Keller Rohrback was the ideal choice. It was an old-line insurance-defense firm, much like his own.

Sarko was surprised to get a call from Bob Piper. He was even more surprised to hear him say he'd soon be stepping in as Foodmaker's new lawyer. Piper told him he'd be taking a very different approach than the one adopted by Foodmaker's current attorney.

"So the stiff-arm tactics will stop?" Sarko asked.

The question felt like a brushback pitch, but Piper didn't flinch. His plan, he assured Sarko, was to abandon the standard adversarial approach that insurance companies typically took and convince Foodmaker to start calling its own shots. That meant doing away with the notion of tricking people into signing away their rights by offering them small checks. Instead, Piper planned to deal equitably with all the poisoned consumers through the class-action. That way, Piper explained, Foodmaker could make good with its customers and go after the meat suppliers that had sent the tainted meat up the food chain.

Sarko liked what he was hearing. "Foodmaker needs to view this as a business problem, not a legal problem," he told Piper.

Piper agreed. But he wanted something in return from Sarko. One of the most immediate threats to Foodmaker's business was the relentless bad press being directed at Jack in the Box. Some of it was being generated by Keller Rohrback lawyers who had taken their fight with David Martin to the newspapers. When he officially took over, Piper wanted this to stop.

Sarko understood. Restaurant chains lived and died on their reputation. Jack in the Box was teetering on complete collapse as its name became increasingly associated with *E. coli*. It wasn't in the interest of Keller Rohrback's clients to see the business go bankrupt.

The two lawyers struck a gentleman's agreement: Sarko promised to shut down all negative press coming out of his office. In return, Piper vowed to do everything in his power to move Foodmaker to deal fairly with all the families that had been injured. Ultimately, he wanted to change the story in the press to "Foodmaker is doing the right thing."

In the back of his mind, Sarko knew that the lawyer saying the most damaging things to the press about Jack in the Box was Bill. More than anything else, Bill's penchant for talking to reporters drove Sarko nuts. True, Bill's media savvy had landed the firm dozens of clients.

But it was time for Sarko to lay down the law with him—no more freewheeling when it came to talking to the press. Going forward, all press interviews regarding the Jack in the Box litigation would have to be cleared by Sarko.

After going through the protocol of calling Sarko and, then Chris Pence, Piper placed a backdoor call to Bill. Piper suspected that Sarko had little to no direct dealings with the clients, that Bill did all that. And Piper wanted a direct channel to the guy talking to the victims and the press.

Besides, he knew Bill. A couple of years earlier they had argued a case against each other. Bill had represented a young Korean girl whose car was broadsided by another vehicle being driven by an executive from one of Seattle's leading telecommunications companies. The executive was driving a company vehicle and was on company time. The company was insured by Chubb, which chose Piper to defend it against the accident claim.

A one-hundred-thousand-dollar policy was in play. The executive claimed the collision was a random accident, and Piper offered to settle for ten thousand dollars. But Bill declined the offer, and the case went to arbitration. Then Bill subpoenaed the telecommunications company and obtained their executive's cell phone records, which showed that the executive had been talking on the phone at the same minute that the accident report indicated the collision had occurred. The implication was clear. The arbitrator awarded all one hundred thousand dollars to Bill's client.

Piper didn't lose many arbitration cases, and Bill's victory earned him instant respect in Piper's eyes, especially since Piper had recommended a personal friend, lawyer George Kargianis, as the arbitrator.

Bill was pleased to get a call from Piper. He had a feeling they'd get along just fine.

Tuesday, March 23, 1993
Seattle Superior Court

Judge Charles Johnson's TRO against Foodmaker and Jack in the Box had become a lightning rod. Normally, a temporary restraining order is just that—temporary. It is a stopgap measure to protect a party facing immediate and irreparable harm. TROs essentially freeze things until a full hearing can be held, enabling both sides to make a case for lifting the order or making it a permanent injunction. They rarely attract press coverage. But in the fourteen days since Johnson had signed the TRO, lawyers on both sides had assumed a take-no-prisoners approach over the outcome. Charges and countercharges of professional misconduct had been levied by the opposing lawyers. Extensive briefs and memos had been filed with the court. Press releases had been issued. It was turning into a sideshow that was overtaking the case itself.

But in many ways the issues raised by the TRO were much more than a sideshow. Rather, the TRO highlighted just how high the stakes had gone. Jack in the Box was caught in the crosshairs of the biggest, most high-profile food poison outbreak in contemporary history. There were more than 650 documented victims in four states. Four children were dead. Many other children were facing lifelong complications. Meanwhile, the nation's fifth-largest fast-food chain was at risk of going under. The company's survival hinged largely on its ability to extinguish the claims of hundreds of injured customers. If the TRO remained in place, Jack in the Box would be forced to settle all the claims through litigation, a much more lengthy and costly process.

The more the spotlight centered on the dispute over the TRO, the more Sarko and Chris Pence seemed to occupy center stage. At least it felt that way to Bill. Sarko and Pence were handling all the court appearances. They were even going out of their way to do press interviews that Bill had set up for himself. In one instance, Sarko and Pence even posed for a newspaper photographer and did a joint interview with a reporter doing a story about how they had ended up working together on the case. Pence called his collaboration with Keller Rohrback "a perfect marriage." It was a marriage arranged by Bill, but he was left completely out of the story.

Meantime, the Karr Tuttle Campbell law firm prepared to take the reins on behalf of Jack in the Box. The judge handling the TRO dispute had scheduled a final hearing on the matter before issuing a ruling. David Martin would be making his final appearance; Bruce Clark would be making his first. The potential for awkwardness was obvious. At the same time, a group of personal-injury lawyers would be hammering away at Jack in the Box for trying to settle on the cheap with injured children. For Clark, it was important to grab control of the situation and send a clear signal to everyone—especially the judge and the opposing lawyers—that a new law firm was in charge. "Let the judge know we are the new sheriff in town and let the plaintiffs' attorneys know they need to be dealing with us," Piper had instructed Clark.

But the message had to be sent without touching off any fireworks. "Just try to make everybody happy," Piper had advised. "The last thing we want is to appear to be picking an ugly fight with the very people we just sickened or killed."

The judge called the parties forward in the *Jack in the Box* case.

"Your Honor, David Martin representing the defendant," Martin began. "I also want to introduce to the Court Mr. Bruce Clark from Karr Tuttle Campbell law firm, who will also be representing Foodmaker, Inc., and will be replacing me as counsel . . . shortly."

That got the judge's attention. "Will be replacing you, as counsel in this case?" the judge asked.

"Yes," Martin said. "The primary carrier has paid out their policy limits. And the excess carrier will be taking over the defense of the lawsuits, and Mr. Clark and his law firm will be assuming the defense. . . . So this is one of my last appearances before Your Honor. You'll probably be pleased with that."

Finally, Clark stepped in.

"Your Honor, may I speak?"

"Well, I'm not sure," the judge said, looking to Martin. "Is he your co-counsel now?"

"Yes he is, Your Honor."

The judge turned to Clark. "Go right ahead."

"Thank you, Your Honor. One reason I wanted to say something is I've already heard some comments . . . about things that have gone on before, of what another insurance company has done. I don't know about that frankly. I know that when my firm arrives in this case there will be a new insurer involved in the case, and frankly what has gone before has no bearing on what will happen henceforth."

Seamlessly, Clark had taken the baton from Martin. By the time the hearing broke up, Piper was mingling with the plaintiffs' lawyers, smiling confidently while tugging on his suspenders with his thumbs as his belly sagged over his belt. With Jack in the Box's $100 million in insurance money about to fall under his control, he had all the leverage. Without saying it, he got his message across to his adversaries: *We're not here to fight. I've been authorized to hand out money.*

22

FOUR-SEASONS JUSTICE

At the end of March, Roni Austin filed a wrongful-death suit against Jack in the Box in Superior Court in San Diego. Bill read a story in the *Seattle Times* reporting that the family of Lauren Rudolph had sued Jack in the Box. "The evidence in our case is irrefutable," attorney Robert Trentacosta was quoted as saying.

An idea popped into Bill's head: *If the outbreak started in San Diego and caused the death of Lauren Rudolph, I should be talking to her attorney.*

He tracked down Trentacosta's number and called him. After a lengthy introductory conversation, Bill invited him up to Seattle. "We should coordinate our efforts," Bill said.

Trentacosta liked the idea and said he'd make travel arrangements.

At the same time, Bill got a message on his voice mail from Piper. "Marler, I can't believe you are stupid enough to have a password that is 1-1-1-1," Piper told him.

Bill stopped to think. It dawned on him that after three years he'd never gotten around to setting his own password. His phone still had the password assigned to it by the factory. As a result, Piper had hacked into his voice mail. Laughing, Bill called him and gave him hell.

Then Piper told him why he had called. Behind the scenes, he had been talking to Jack in the Box officials and had convinced them that the company's interests would be far better served by hiring a private judge to focus exclusively on their case. The idea made a lot of sense. Judges have lots of cases on their dockets, a fact of life that makes the wheels of justice turn slowly at the courthouse. This worked against Jack in the Box's interests. The company needed to put the outbreak in the rearview mirror as soon as possible. Ideally, that meant moving the class-action litigation outside the courts altogether and finding a nonjudicial vehicle, such as having a special master preside over the case.

Washington law had a provision that authorized the presiding judge in a lawsuit to appoint a special master—often known as a judge pro tempore—to come in from the outside to preside exclusively over a single complex case. Piper had just the man in mind—retired judge

Judge Terrence Carroll was appointed by a judge to be a special master presiding over the Jack in the Box litigation.

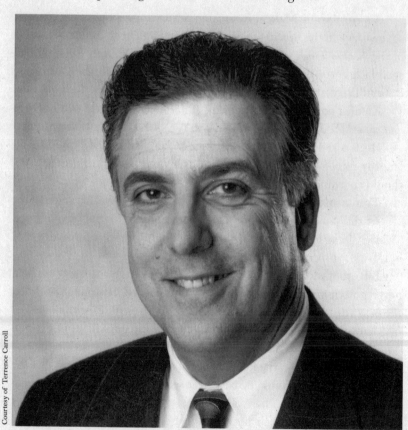

Terrence Carroll. Judge Carroll had been a distinguished Superior Court judge who recently left the bench to join a private mediation and arbitration firm. More important, Piper knew and trusted him.

It all sounded good to Jack in the Box. But before the court would go along with it, Piper was going to need Keller Rohrback to endorse the plan. Bill assured him he was on board. Bill knew Judge Carroll well. He had presided over the air-disaster trial that Bill had worked on in his first year out of law school. Bill told Piper that he expected Sarko would go along with the idea of hiring Carroll.

Sarko was intrigued when Piper called to propose hiring a private judge to adjudicate their case. The concept wasn't new to Sarko. When big corporations ended up in high-stakes legal disputes it wasn't unusual for them to hire a private judge, enabling them to avoid the congested court system and receive the undivided attention of a presiding magistrate. Sarko liked to think of it as "four seasons justice." But the *Jack in the Box* case wasn't commercial litigation between two corporate titans. Rather, hundreds of children and their parents were suing a company. In that respect, Piper's idea was a novel one.

One aspect of the idea appealed to Sarko right away—his clients would get to zip past the hundreds of other people whose cases were ahead of them in the King County court system's docket. Plus, Judge Terry Carroll had a great reputation for competence and fairness.

But Sarko had worked on commercial cases where private judges were hired. It was a very expensive process. Typically, the cost for a private judge was split between the two parties. When Sarko raised the cost factor, Piper acknowledged that even with Carroll at the helm the case could take a couple of years to resolve and Carroll wouldn't come cheap.

Sarko couldn't help wondering if this were a trap. A typical defense strategy was to grind a plaintiff into the ground by outspending the opponent. Certainly Foodmaker and Jack in the Box had far more resources at their disposal than the families of poisoned children did.

"Of course, you're paying," Sarko said.

"Of course," Piper said.

Now, that's unique, Sarko thought, now convinced that Piper was sincere about getting the claims resolved as quickly and painlessly as possible.

Sarko agreed to join Piper in asking the court to appoint Terry Carroll as a special master to preside over the *Jack in the Box* class-action case, and on April 22, 1993, Judge Charles Johnson signed an order declaring Judge Terry Carroll was judge pro tempore in the *Jack in the Box* class-action case.

But Piper was surprised when he picked up a copy of the morning paper and saw a story reporting that Jack in the Box and lawyers for injured children had agreed to have an outside judge preside over their case. He knew he hadn't talked to the press and neither had Jack in the Box officials. That meant someone from Keller Rohrback had, and Piper didn't appreciate it. On something like this, nobody should have gone to the media without his approval. Piper felt it made him look bad in the eyes of his client; it seemed he wasn't in total control.

Piper suspected Bill was behind this. He and Bill had been talking about doing a joint press release, but clearly Bill had gotten ahead of him on this.

A master manipulator, Piper telephoned Sarko, who was in a conference room when the receptionist put Piper's call through. There was no hello. Piper just ripped into Sarko and accused him of violating their agreement.

Sarko was blindsided. At first he had no idea what Piper was ranting about. He hadn't had a chance to look at the morning paper. But by the time the conversation was winding down, Sarko knew why Piper was so uptight. He was also pretty sure he knew who had talked to the media—Bill. Sarko apologized profusely to Piper, hung up the phone, went down to Bill's office, and exploded.

"What the f—— is going on?" he demanded and launched into a rant about his call from Piper.

Bill gave him a puzzled look. He acknowledged having talked to the press, but he didn't understand all the fuss. It wasn't as if both sides hadn't agreed to a private judge.

Sarko said he wasn't there to debate the issue. He was sick and tired of Bill's freewheeling, particularly when it came to the press. Now

Sarko had egg on his face in Piper's eyes. It was high time Bill started following the chain of command in the law firm. Sarko stormed out.

Bill didn't appreciate being scolded like a teenager who had just broken curfew. Since the start of the outbreak he'd invested countless hours studying the science of *E. coli* in order to position himself as an authority on the subject. As a result the media routinely called him with questions and the firm frequently got mentioned in the press. The visibility Bill had generated was a big part of the reason Keller Rohrback had well over fifty clients from the outbreak. No other firm had close to that. It didn't seem that Sarko appreciated that fact.

Denis Stearns looked on in amazement as Piper nimbly went from screaming at Sarko to dialing up the PR people at Jack in the Box in San Diego and speaking in a relaxed, confident tone as he told them about the story in the paper and assured them that it said everything he wanted it to say. Things were moving along according to plan. Everything was under control.

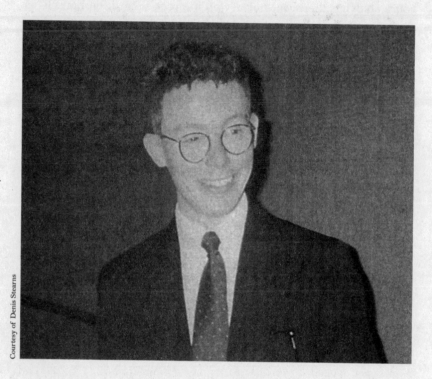

Denis Stearns was Bob Piper's young protégé and handled the discovery process during the litigation.

23

MIRROR, MIRROR ON THE WALL

No one would come out and admit it, but some internal tension had emerged over who was in control of the Jack in the Box litigation at Keller Rohrback. Sarko was the managing partner, and he and Pence were stepping into all the high-profile moments of the case. But Bill was the driving force behind the scenes—reeling in the clients, lining up the experts, and maintaining the ever-important relationship with Piper. It seemed to Bill that he and Griffin were doing all the grunt work while getting pushed aside by Sarko and Pence whenever it was time to go to court or talk to the press. That didn't seem to bother Griffin—he was the ultimate team player. But Bill chafed under this approach.

The thing that annoyed him the most was the sense that Sarko and Pence looked down on him for being a media hound. Sarko had already made it clear to Bill that he didn't want him or anyone else talking to the press on the *Jack in the Box* case without clearing it first. Bill interpreted the real purpose behind this as an effort to keep him in his place. He couldn't help believing that the other guys, if given the opportunity, would talk to the media without getting clearance.

He decided to test his theory by having a little fun. He telephoned Chris Pence's office and told the receptionist that he was a producer for *The Oprah Winfrey Show*. He asked the receptionist to give Mr. Pence the message that Oprah wanted to interview him in connection with a show she was planning on *E. coli*. Bill told the receptionist he'd call back later that day to discuss the interview with Pence. At the appointed time, Bill called back, and Pence eagerly jumped on the line, ready to talk to *The Oprah Winfrey Show*. "Hey Chris, it's Marler. Gotcha!" he said, laughing wildly as Pence swore at him.

April 30, 1993

"I love you, Mommy." Those were the first words Brianne whispered after starting to regain her speech. Doctors informed Suzanne that it would take some time before Brianne said much beyond that. She had suffered two strokes that had impaired her speech capabilities, among other things. She'd also had a breathing tube down her throat for forty days, which did a number on her vocal cords. It would be a couple of weeks more before she would be strong enough to begin working with a speech therapist.

Looking at her daughter, Suzanne tried to keep a stiff upper lip. But it wasn't easy. The doctors did their best to explain that there was a long, rough road ahead. Brianne had survived HUS, but it was going to require another miracle for her to return to some semblance of normalcy. All her hair had fallen out. Most of her large intestine had been removed. Her kidneys and liver had suffered permanent damage. Those were some of the physical problems. The damage to her brain produced another set of challenges. Her cognitive motor skills had been severely compromised. She'd have to relearn basic things like how to read, write, walk, bathe, and brush her teeth.

Suzanne had a hard time coming to grips with it all. *How long would this go on for?*

Doctors were predicting that Brianne would be strong enough to begin rehabilitation therapy in about two weeks. In the meantime, she would remain at the hospital under the care of nurses and specialists.

Suzanne hadn't been home in over six weeks. But she planned to remain at the hospital and be there to hold Brianne's hand through the duration of the rehabilitation process. Meantime, she was getting totally overwhelmed by the thought of everything else going on around her: endless paperwork from the hospital and the insurance company, home finances that had been neglected for four months, and constant media inquiries about her daughter's progress. Aside from Brianne's health, the biggest source of anxiety was the skyrocketing hospitalization bill and the upcoming rehab costs. Then there would be long-term, in-home care. Increasingly, Suzanne felt the need to secure an attorney to help her recover costs from Jack in the Box.

Mike Canaan had arranged times for each of the attorneys on his list to meet with Suzanne at the hospital. But he'd also done some additional research on his own and noticed that Keller Rohrback surfaced in more news stories than any other firm since the start of the outbreak. Yet no attorney from that firm was on the short list approved by Suzanne's brother, Garry. On his own, Canaan called Keller Rohrback and asked to speak to the lawyer in charge of the *Jack in the Box* case.

The receptionist put the call through to Bill Marler.

"This is Bill."

Canaan was surprised. The voice sounded so . . . young. All the lawyers that he had called were considerably older. Bill sounded more down-to-earth, too. Canaan liked that. He identified himself and his affiliation to the Kiner family. Then he explained that he was calling lawyers and assembling a short list of candidates to represent the family, from which the Kiners would select one.

Bill had never had a private investigator call him on behalf of a prospective client before. Intrigued, Bill asked Canaan about his background. Canaan started with his time in the Marine Corps as a security officer aboard the White House helicopter.

"My dad is a marine," Bill said, having been drilled that once a marine, always a marine, even in retirement.

Just like that, they began swapping military stories.

Canaan warmed up to Bill fast. He liked Bill even more once he started talking about Jack in the Box and its culpability in the *E. coli* outbreak. Bill's knowledge of the pathogen was impressive, too, particularly of how it impacted children. Bill no longer sounded like the folksy young lawyer who had answered the phone; he sounded like a take-charge attorney on a mission.

Canaan had heard enough. He promised to get back to Bill soon.

Later that day, Canaan met with Suzanne. She was holding the list of prospective lawyers that her brother wanted her to meet. "Is there anyone that you'd like to see added to this list?" she asked.

"Yes," Canaan said.

"Who?"

"Bill Marler."

Suzanne had never heard the name, but if Canaan suggested him, that was good enough for her.

"Why don't you arrange for him to meet me here at the hospital?" she said. "I'd like to meet with him alone."

Bill had been over Bob Nugent's congressional testimony numerous times. He was particularly drawn to the exchanges over Jack in the Box's failure to cook its hamburgers to Washington's 155-degree requirement. "We were not aware of the Washington State regulation," Nugent had testified.

That assertion had never made sense to Bill. It just didn't ring true. When your business is selling hamburgers, Bill reasoned, there's no excuse for not being aware of the latest laws and regulations governing its safety. He was unaware that Jack in the Box's internal investigation had found two notices in its files from county health departments in Washington. Nor did Bill know about the admission that Nugent had made to his shareholders, or that it had been reported in an industry publication. But even if Bill had known about those things, none of this would have changed his gut feeling that decision-makers at Jack in the Box had known about the temperature-change regulation and chosen to ignore it because it was higher than all the other states where Jack in the Box did business. Big fast-food chains loved uniformity. It was much simpler to produce one operations manual with cooking guidelines for all cooks in all restaurants, regardless of what state they worked in.

Entitled to get at Jack in the Box's internal documents and memos through the discovery process, Bill fired off a slew of requests for production—formal requests for company records. He wanted every manual, memo, and document that related to the storage, preparation, cooking, and handling of meat.

The requests ultimately landed in the hands of Denis Stearns. Bill's allegation that people had purposely ignored food-safety rules rubbed him the wrong way. *Where does this SOB get off making that kind of claim?*

Stearns planned to make Bill work for the information he was after. The rules governing document requests under discovery called for specificity. Before Bill saw anything, he was going to need to clean up his request. Meantime, Stearns discussed the situation with Piper.

Privy to more information than Stearns, Piper knew about the notices that had surfaced in Jack in the Box's files and that Nugent had pinned blame on Ken Dunkley for the oversight. But something about that scenario troubled Piper: it felt too convenient. After all, Jack in the Box was the fifth-largest fast-food chain in the U.S. In Washington alone it had sixty-six restaurants. If the state was so concerned about *E. coli* and the need to raise cooking temperatures in meat, why hadn't the company turned up more than a couple of obscure notices from county health departments? And if the new regulation had been in effect for almost a year before the outbreak, why in the hell wasn't the state aware that one of the biggest chains in its jurisdiction wasn't in compliance?

Piper didn't know the answers. But he had a hunch where to look to get them. He gave Stearns another assignment: "Find out everything there is to know about the state regulations."

Stearns jotted down notes as Piper fired off questions.

"Just because the state board of health passed the regulation, does it automatically apply in every county?" Piper asked. "And how are the counties notified?"

Piper reminded Stearns to draft a detailed memo documenting his findings.

Stearns snickered. Piper was a master at creating billable hours. As the case continued to pick up steam, the firm had been pressuring him to raise his hourly rate. But Piper consistently refused. "It's not the rate that matters," he told Stearns. "It's how many hours you bill."

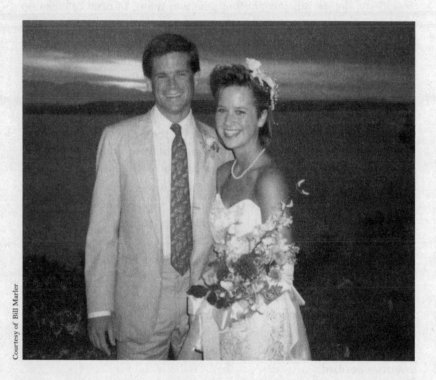

Julie and Bill Marler married shortly after she had overcome cancer and he had gone through a painful divorce.

24

A TOTAL LONG SHOT

Early May 1993

"HEY, HONEY," BILL SHOUTED AS HE CAME THROUGH THE DOOR. "YOU'LL never believe who I got a call from today."

"Who?"

"The Brianne Kiner family."

"You're kidding."

Bill laughed.

"They called *you*?" she said.

"I'm meeting with Mrs. Kiner at the hospital tomorrow."

"Honey, that's fantastic."

"Yeah, but they'll never hire me," he said, becoming more serious. The other lawyers under consideration were far more established. The fact that Mrs. Kiner's brother was an established lawyer didn't bode well either. He'd undoubtedly be more partial toward a more experienced, big-name plaintiffs' lawyer. Bill fully appreciated that way of thinking.

Julie couldn't help thinking that if Bill actually got to talk to the family he'd win them over.

"It's a total long shot," he said.

That night Julie didn't fall asleep easily. Her mind was on Bill's meeting with Brianne Kiner. It was the kind of opportunity that came along only once. He had to make a good first impression. That got her thinking about the first impression Bill had made on her.

In the summer of 1986 Bill was a depressed twenty-nine-year-old law student who was separated from his wife but not yet divorced. At the time, he was clerking at a downtown law firm where Julie worked as a receptionist fielding upward of sixty calls per hour. She was twenty and had alluring eyes and a warm smile. Yet she was self-conscious. She'd put on twenty-five pounds in a few months' time. It felt like even more on her 5'4" frame. She started dressing differently. But even loosely fitting clothes couldn't hide her puffy cheeks. Lucky for her, the lawyers ignored the receptionist as long as she properly directed the calls and efficiently sorted the mail.

In between calls one afternoon, Julie looked up and discovered a visitor peering over the reception counter. "Hi," he said, offering a polite smile. "I'm Bill Marler."

She knew him as the cute law clerk that always buzzed around with a purposeful look in his eyes. But a few months earlier something had changed. The other receptionist reported rumors that Bill's wife had left him.

"Hello," she said, smiling nervously. "I'm Julie . . . Julie Dueck."

Bill observed Julie's punk haircut. Her head was shaved, except for a few long strands. Cool if you hang out in Seattle's university district. But a bit bold for the reception area of a conservative law firm.

"Nice hairdo," Bill said sarcastically.

Her smile melted. "I'm going through chemotherapy and radiation, and my hair is falling out."

Bill's jaw dropped. "Oh."

Embarrassed, he took a couple of steps back and scurried off. Later, after Julie had left for the day, Bill cornered the other receptionist. She confirmed that Julie had non-Hodgkin's lymphoma and was on an aggressive treatment schedule that included cancer-killing drugs and regular radiation treatments. That, explained the receptionist, was why Julie sometimes wore an ice cap—a turban packed with ice—atop her head. Bill had never noticed. He felt like an idiot.

When Julie got to work the next day, a brand-new teddy bear outfitted in a white sweater and a blue bow tie was waiting for her at the reception desk. A card wished her good luck with her remaining chemo and radiation treatments. It was signed "Bill Marler."

Julie was stunned. On one level, it felt like the kind of gift a girl might get from a protective older brother. But the bear symbolized something more for her—recognition. Other than her fellow receptionist, no one at the firm ever talked to Julie, especially about her cancer. From then on she brought the bear along to every treatment.

Several months later Bill's divorce was finalized, and he started seeing Julie. At first, they were two friends helping each other through tough times. Nine years separated them. But her cancer and his divorce brought them closer together.

Eventually they fell in love and got married. To Julie, the teddy bear with the white sweater and blue bow tie symbolized the start of the best thing that had ever happened to her—marrying Bill Marler. That was why she held on to it all these years.

The next morning, Bill was up, dressed and headed for the door very early. He had a lot of work to do before heading over to the hospital. "Hey Jules, I'll see you tonight," he hollered over his shoulder.

"Wait," she yelled from the bedroom. Moments later she met him at the front door and handed him the teddy bear. He hadn't seen it in years. But he recognized it instantly. It brought to his mind the sight of Julie without any hair, and then the beginning of their relationship.

"You should give this to Brianne," Julie said

Bill paused, realizing what this bear meant to Julie. He looked her in the eye, as if to ask, *Are you sure?*

A smile slowly crept across her face.

He stuffed the bear in his duffle bag, kissed Julie's lips, and headed for the ferry. He couldn't help thinking that the best decision he had ever made was marrying her.

Later, at the office, Bill told a couple of colleagues that he was going to meet with Brianne Kiner's mother. They agreed that this was significant. A good first impression could go a long way to securing the Kiner family as a client for the firm. They were eager to hear the outcome.

Bill hadn't talked to Sarko about the meeting. Sarko had a strong aversion to associates' meeting alone with potential clients. He preferred a partner to go along, especially in a situation where the stakes were as high as they were in the *Kiner* case. Bill knew how Sarko felt, but taking a partner along wasn't a written policy. Besides, Bill felt perfectly capable of handling the meeting alone.

Mike Canaan picked Bill up at his law firm late in the morning and drove him to the hospital. It was Bill's first time inside Children's Hospital. They made their way to the fourth floor and entered the ICU. Unsure of what to expect, Bill took a deep breath and entered Brianne's room.

Brianne was lying on the bed, her eyes shut. Bandages covered large portions of her upper body. Wires, cords, and tubes connected her to an IV bag and an array of beeping machines. She had just come off dialysis, and her white skin had turned dark brown and leathery— showing the effects of her kidneys' being shut down for so long. She had lost most of her large intestine, and doctors were preparing to reconnect her bowel.

Suzanne immediately stood up. Wearing a double-extra-large black T-shirt with a giant Mickey Mouse emblazoned on it, and wrinkled black cotton pants, she looked like a woman badly in need of sleep and an ironing board. Her arms waving, she talked fast and started firing off questions.

Bill missed most of what she said, distracted by the shock of seeing Brianne. He couldn't take his eyes off her. Her appearance reminded him of a mummy in a natural history museum—shriveled, brittle, and haunting.

Suzanne kept talking, and her voice getting louder and more animated.

Then the pile of bandages moved and Brianne opened her eyes. "M-ahhh-mmm . . ." she cried in a high-pitched, guttural voice. "Ssss-tttt-ah-ppp . . . it."

Bill's eyes enlarged as he backed up slowly until he hit the wall behind him. Tears welled up. Brianne's voice sounded ancient. He'd never heard anything so feeble. He'd never seen anything so pathetic.

Suzanne quit talking.

Brianne closed her eyes again.

Everything stopped but the beeping machines.

Speechless, Bill stumbled into the hallway. He'd been reading all the literature on *E. coli* and he'd been talking to medical experts, but nothing had prepared him for the sight of a little girl so ravaged by a foodborne illness. It was hard to comprehend that all this damage could be the result of taking a few bites out of a hamburger. Staring at the ceiling, he thought of his daughter, Morgan. What if this happened to her? How would he react? What would he do? How would he feel?

He wiped his eyes, trying to pull himself together.

Suzanne was waiting for him beside Brianne when Bill stepped back into the room. She looked at his eyes, red and blinking rapidly.

"I'm very sorry," he whispered.

Suzanne explained just how profound Brianne's injuries had been.

Bill just listened for nearly an hour. Then, before leaving, Bill handed Suzanne the teddy bear. "It's for Brianne," he said.

Suzanne could tell the bear wasn't brand-new. She sensed there was a story behind it.

Bill gestured to invite Suzanne to step into the hallway with him. There he told her about Julie and her bout with cancer at a young age. The bear, Bill explained, was something he had given Julie to help get her through the ordeal.

Her emotions already close to the surface, Suzanne started to cry. As a mother, she picked up on something subtle about Bill right away: *This guy is sensitive enough to tell me this outside the earshot of Brianne.* She thanked Bill for coming.

Mike Canaan was out in the hallway, waiting to drive Bill back to his law office. But Bill told Canaan he'd find his own way back to his law office. He needed time alone to think.

More than anything, he now wanted to go to bat for Brianne and Suzanne Kiner.

Before meeting them, Bill's priority had been to position the firm to land Brianne as a client. But as soon as he saw Brianne, something changed inside him. She was no longer a prospective client; she was a daughter fighting for her life. Bill couldn't help putting himself in Suzanne's shoes and wondering what kind of shape he'd be in if that had been his daughter, Morgan, lying on the hospital bed, cut open, and connected to machines.

He knew he was acting precisely the way a lawyer was trained not to act. Only he wasn't acting. That was the problem.

One senior lawyer had insisted on accompanying Bill to the meeting, but Bill had insisted on going alone. Maybe he should have listened to the guy with more experience.

By the time he reached his office the redness had left his eyes and he put on an expression of confidence. He had to figure out what he was going to tell the partners. They would be expecting a report on his visit.

"So how did it go?" one of the partners asked.

Bill explained that the Kiners had talked to numerous firms. But now the family was thinking seriously about Keller Rohrback. "We have a great chance of getting the case," he told them.

The minute Bill walked through the door that night Julie knew something was wrong. She could read him like a book. "Honey, what happened?"

"I blew it. I went into the room and I just couldn't . . ."

He tilted his head back and took a deep breath. The tears were too close to the surface to hold back.

Julie waited.

"You'll never believe what this little girl has gone through. It's completely unimaginable that something she ate can cause something so catastrophic."

Even as he graphically described Brianne's injuries, Julie had trouble imagining the picture he was painting.

"It has turned the family's world upside down," he said. "I just don't know how this family is functioning."

The only time Julie had seen Bill cry this way was back before they were dating, when he was going through his divorce.

"This could happen to our daughter," Bill said softly. "This could be Morgan."

25

I DON'T MEAN TO BE IMPOLITE

Bob Nugent hated to do it, but he had to let Jody Powell go. Jack in the Box was bleeding money, and it couldn't afford Powell's rate of eighty thousand dollars per week. Revenue had dropped off a cliff. Most menu items had been reduced to one dollar in an attempt to attract people back to the restaurants. To a degree, it was working, but Nugent knew he was losing money by the day.

Nonetheless, Nugent was encouraged by Dave Theno's progress on the food-safety front. He had begun rolling out his revolutionary food-inspection system. It didn't take long for meat suppliers to realize that if they wanted to supply frozen patties to one of the largest hamburger chains in the U.S., there were new rules, starting at the slaughterhouses.

Theno distributed a checklist that specified skinning techniques (cuts through the side only, pulling without contamination), carcass washing and bacteriocidal treatment (water-temperature and pressure guidelines, acid concentration), evisceration splitting (no intestinal breakage, viscera-inspection program, and sterilizers), hot box/coolers (spray chill system, carcass-temperature drops, and contamination control), and fabrication (carcass-temperature control, fabrication-room sanitization, micro profiling, employee practices, and knife sterilizers).

Jack in the Box's new requirements for the meat-grinding and -packing plants was just as stringent, starting with a full-scale inspection of raw materials the minute they arrived from the slaughterhouses. From there, a certain product temperature had to be maintained and

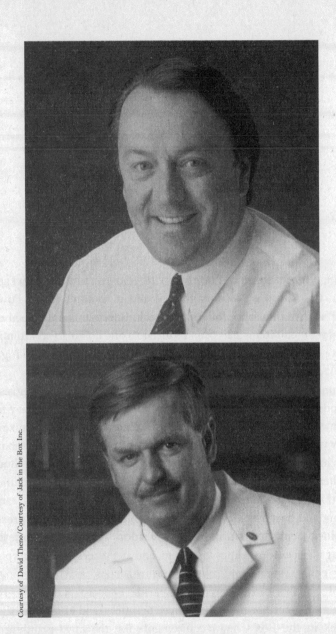

Courtesy of David Theno/Courtesy of Jack in the Box Inc.

Bob Nugent (top) and Dave Theno (bottom) instituted the toughest food-safety standards in the fast-food industry after the E. coli *outbreak.*

all products had to be assigned lot numbers and tracking numbers. At each step—blending and fat adjustment, patty forming, freezing and casing—the highest sanitation and handling procedures were expected.

"The government doesn't require all this," one plant executive complained to Theno.

"You know what?" Theno said. "I don't really give a shit what the government requires."

From Theno's perspective, the most telling aspect of his new guidelines was the microbial profiling he required on the part of the grinding and patty-making facility. These were the last guys to handle the meat before it was trucked to the restaurants for sale to consumers. The tests that Theno had them administer tracked the total amount of bacteria in beef patties, along with specific counts for *Listeria*, *Salmonella*, and *E. coli* O157:H7.

A pound has 454 grams. When Theno first started demanding tests from the meat plants, the initial results indicated the presence of 100,000 to 300,000 organisms of generic *E. coli* per gram of beef. Theno showed those results to Nugent.

"We are finding *E. coli* at a rate of about five samples per one thousand tests," Theno said. "That's about one-half of one percent."

The number didn't mean anything to Nugent.

Theno said simply that these levels were way higher than anyone in the beef industry expected. Way higher!

Nugent asked what the industry estimated as the percentage of *E. coli* in meat at the time.

"Hundredths of a percent, maybe," Theno said.

Nugent understood that number. The difference between 0.5 percent and 0.01 percent was huge, particularly when dealing with a bacterial pathogen.

The good news was that the test results were enabling Jack in the Box to identify which plants were willing to implement Theno's new safety protocols. The plants whose meat showed a continual drop in the percentage of *E. coli* organisms in a gram of beef were the ones the restaurant chain would do business with. Period.

Meat suppliers and slaughterhouses weren't the only ones in an uproar over Theno's new approach. One afternoon Theno got a call from the head of the National Council of Chain Restaurants (NCCR). All of the big chains—McDonald's, Taco Bell, Burger King—were represented by NCCR. The director had been hearing a lot of feedback throughout the industry on Theno's new food-safety protocols at Jack in the Box. Beef suppliers were complaining about the cost. Product development guys argued that taste would be compromised. And some of Jack in the Box's competitors was apprehensive about how the system might force them to change. Theno knew the director well.

"Dave, I'm just calling to give you a head's up," she said. "This whole meat-sampling program you're talking about isn't making some of our friends very happy."

Theno listened politely for a few minutes until he'd heard enough.

"Well, last Wednesday when my paycheck came, it had a Jack in the Box logo in the corner," he said. "So that's who I'm supposed to take care of. So I don't mean to be impolite, but next time your friends call, tell them to go screw themselves."

The director was speechless.

"And another thing," Theno continued. "If they have an issue with Dave Theno, you tell them to call my ass. They know how to find me. Now I'm not doing this to piss them off. I'm doing this because we have to. So I don't really give a shit what they think."

Theno hung up the phone.

26

IN YOUR FACE

SUZANNE KINER WAS SMART. BUT NO ONE HAD EVER TOLD HER THAT. When she was growing up, her brother was always the smart one. Naturally, he went on to become the lawyer. Suzanne had wanted to go into medicine, but she had ended up being a full-time mother instead. She knew she wasn't the family expert on law, but she was confident she knew more about her children's needs than anyone. And she was convinced that what Brianne needed most in a lawyer was a young, hungry lion.

She looked at the piece of paper in her hand and reviewed the names of the five candidates that her brother had chosen for her. She'd now met with each of them. All were highly qualified. None were young and hungry like Bill Marler. She called her brother to discuss her preference.

Hubert was adamant that any one of the top two or three names on the list Canaan had generated would be ideal for Brianne. When Suzanne tried to make a case for hiring Bill, Hubert pushed back. He was experienced enough to tell that that Bill wasn't experienced enough. The depth of Brianne's injuries and the lack of understanding regarding *E. coli* guaranteed that the case would be complicated at many levels. The family didn't need a lawyer who would be undergoing on-the-job training. They needed a trial lawyer with a track record of handling big cases. He reminded Suzanne that Bill was at the beginning of his career while these others were at the zenith of theirs. On paper the choice was clear.

But Suzanne made decisions based on feelings and intuition. *E. coli* was a very unconventional pathogen that had invaded Brianne through the most innocent thing a child does: eating. It was going to take an unconventional approach to get the kind of justice Suzanne was after. "I nearly lost my daughter over corporate greed," she explained. "I want to make it my mission to make meat safety an in-your-face issue. I'm not going to go quiet."

She believed Bill Marler wasn't going to go quietly either.

Hubert was focused on compensation, not political advocacy.

But for the entire time that Brianne was confined to a bed in the ICU, Suzanne was tethered to her side. For much of that time Brianne was on a respirator while a machine was enabling her heart to beat at a rate of six times per minute. If that machine missed its rhythm just once, Suzanne noticed it. *E. coli* had changed Suzanne because it had changed her little girl. She wanted a lawyer who understood that.

"I wanted someone who could come in and spend fifteen minutes just absorbing her," Suzanne explained. "Bill was the only one that could look at her. The other ones glanced and then focused only on me. They couldn't look at her."

Late May 1993

"I have Suzanne Kiner on the line for you."

The receptionist's words froze Bill. He hadn't expected to hear from her again. If anything, he had figured Mike Canaan would be calling to let him know that another attorney had been selected.

Bill took the call.

"Can you come back to the hospital?" Suzanne said.

Bill dropped everything and went right over. They met in the lobby. Suzanne was wearing the same clothes she had had on three days earlier. Bill recommended they go somewhere for lunch, and they settled on a nearby Chinese restaurant.

Over the next two hours Suzanne walked Bill through the horrible details of Brianne's ordeal. Bill never touched his food. And he never glanced at his watch.

Suzanne noticed things like that.

Finally she shared the terrible dilemma she had faced over the decision to remove Brianne from life support. "Brianne was brain dead," she began and then paused. Recounting the doctor's words was difficult. "He had told me," Suzanne recalled, "Brianne could not think, hear, smell, or know someone's touch."

The family was faced with the decision whether to remove Brianne from life support.

In trying to recount those dark hours, Suzanne struggled. "I'm sensitive," she whimpered.

Bill hadn't realized how close Suzanne had come to pulling the plug. "Oh, we came so close," said Suzanne.

He could only begin to imagine how agonizing that must have been. But after spending nearly two hours listening to Suzanne vent,

---

Bill Marler had far less experience than any of the lawyers interviewed by the Kiner family. But he was the only one that Suzanne Kiner wanted to represent Brianne.

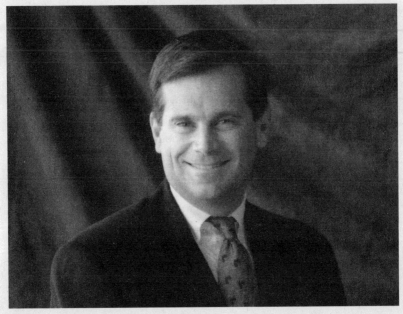

Courtesy of Bill Marler

he began to sense that she was about to endure a lot more stress and anguish. Brianne had finally regained enough strength to start rehab. It would be weeks, if not longer, before she was capable of being discharged from the hospital. But at that stage, Brianne would require full in-home, round-the-clock nursing care. A medical team would have to be assembled to monitor her condition, administer a myriad of medications, and put her through daily courses of rehabilitation. A case manager had to be selected to oversee all of this. Plus, it would take a full-time clerk to manage all of the paperwork, insurance forms, and medical bills.

Suzanne took a deep breath. It was all so overwhelming, so intimidating.

The anxiety in her voice was palpable. Bill encouraged her to just focus on Brianne. He promised he'd help her with the rest.

Reassured, Suzanne said goodbye to Bill. Then she remembered one more thing she had meant to tell him: she'd given the teddy bear to Brianne and told her the story behind it, and Brianne had decided to give the bear a name.

"That's great," Bill said. "What did she name it?"

"Uncle Bill," Suzanne whispered softly, holding back tears.

Bill didn't know what to say.

When Bill got home from work that night, he had that look in his eye. Julie didn't know quite how to describe it. But she had first seen it back when she decided to start dating Bill. Julie's father—a zealous Mennonite with strong convictions about morality and religion—violently opposed her getting involved with a divorced lawyer who was nine years older than she was and who didn't practice religion. To him, that was akin to marrying a heathen. When Julie tried explaining that they were simply dating, her father ordered her to cut off the relationship. When Julie refused, he threatened Julie with physical violence and ultimately shunned her, casting her out of the family. Overnight, Julie was cut off from her entire support system. Her plight seemed to flip a switch in Bill. First he helped her obtain a restraining order against her father. Then he helped her relocate from her college apartment in Bellingham to a place in Seattle near the University of Washington, where he helped her enroll. He got her a good job working for a friend of his in the city. He even negotiated with the clinic and hospital where Julie had been treated for cancer, working out an agreement that enabled Julie to pay off her medical bills a little at a time, since her father would no longer be paying. The more Bill helped Julie the more committed they became to each other.

The Kiners' situation had tripped that switch in Bill. He couldn't stop thinking about their dilemma. The family hadn't officially settled on a lawyer yet. But to Bill's way of thinking, the fact that he hadn't been retained—or that the family hadn't yet gotten around to suing Jack in the Box—shouldn't prevent them from getting money to cover their mounting medical expenses. To Bill, those responsible for having sold contaminated food ought to step up and do the right thing on the front end. By doing so, Jack in the Box wouldn't just demonstrate good faith; it would be a way for restaurant chain to show that it really cared about its customers. More important, Brianne needed assistance now. The family couldn't afford to wait for the legal process to play out. Nor should they have to.

Of course there was zero precedent for what Bill had in mind. But he decided to pay Bob Piper a visit.

Piper couldn't figure out why the Kiner family still hadn't hired a lawyer. What the hell was taking so long? He'd gotten wind that the family had been talking to some of the biggest personal-injury firms in the city. By this point Piper figured that one of these firms would have contacted him about the case. But he hadn't heard a peep. It was odd.

Denis Stearns agreed.

Then Stearns learned that Bill Marler was in the lobby, asking to see Piper. They figured he was there to discuss the class-action. Piper invited him in.

Trying to ignore the seductive glance of the naked woman framed on Piper's wall, Bill sat down and said he was there to discuss Brianne Kiner. He gave Piper a heads-up on her medical situation. Piper appreciated the update, particularly the information about Brianne's eventual release from the hospital. The media would surely make a spectacle out of the event and Piper liked knowing ahead of time so he could apprise his clients.

Then Bill got to the real purpose of his visit. Suzanne hadn't been home in months. She'd essentially been living at the hospital. As a result, the house needed some serious professional cleaning. But the family didn't have the money.

More important, once Brianne got home she would require in-home health care, including nurses and a case manager. These were significant costs and the family didn't have insurance to cover them.

Piper sensed where this was heading—Bill wanted Jack in the Box to pay for all of this. Yet Bill didn't represent the Kiner family and the Kiner family hadn't sued Jack in the Box. This posed a number of problems. Technically, Bill didn't have the authority to seek payment from Jack in the Box on behalf of the Kiners. On the other hand, there was nothing prohibiting Jack in the Box from volunteering to help Brianne. Piper liked the idea. He thought it was exactly the kind of thing Jack in the Box ought to be doing.

The bigger problem was going to be convincing the insurance companies to go along with the plan. Insurers didn't pay for things prior to a final settlement. There really was no precedent for what Bill was seeking. For this to work, ultimately Jack in the Box was going to have to convince its insurers to play along.

Even though the whole scenario was unorthodox, Piper liked it because his primary goal was to do anything and everything to keep the *Kiner* case from becoming a lawsuit. So anything that created a positive vibe between his client and the family was a good thing. He'd figure out how to convince Jack in the Box and its insurers to go along with it later. He gave Bill the green light to have the Kiners' house professionally cleaned and to hire health care professionals to take care of Brianne.

"Have them send the bills to me," Piper said.

27

BABY STEPS

Brianne Kiner couldn't wait to go home. Suzanne couldn't wait either. The staff at Children's Hospital understood. But there was a long way to go before that could happen. First, she had to learn to walk again.

Seated in a wheelchair with a hospital band around her wrist, Brianne waited for her physical therapist. Wearing glasses, a white T-shirt, and purple gym shorts, she was dressed like any other ten-year-old. But her body didn't fit the clothes. Her legs were spindly, making her tennis shoes look three times too big. The hair on the top of her head still hadn't regenerated, giving her the appearance of an elderly woman. Yet she had a smile on her face. Her atrophied muscles were slowly regaining strength. Her limbs weren't as stiff as they had been. Her hand-to-eye coordination was starting to return.

The therapist helped her out of the wheelchair and onto a padded mat. Brianne lay down on her right side. Slowly, the therapist helped her raise her left leg. Up and down, Brianne repeated the regimen. Then she rolled over to her right side and repeated the exercise with her right leg. The exercises were designed to increase her range of motion and flexibility.

Once those were finished, the therapist had Brianne lie on her back, her head resting on a pillow. She bent her knees and pulled her legs up toward her waist. The therapist then knelt down on the pad. With Brianne's feet between the therapist's legs, the therapist placed her hands on the outside of Brianne's knees and told her to try to push her legs outward. The resistance of the therapist's hands caused Brianne to strain. But the therapist encouraged her, telling her she was doing a great job.

The sessions were long and tedious. But Brianne was a quiet fighter. She never complained. She never quit. And she seemed to understand that the public had taken a great interest in her recovery.

When the hospital informed her that one of the city's top television personalities wanted to interview her about the rehabilitation process, Brianne agreed. One day after a therapy session, Brianne met the newscaster in her hospital room. After conducting the interview, the newscaster gave Brianne a gift. It was a children's book about a young girl who wanted to become a ballerina. She offered to read Brianne the story. Brianne liked that.

When the story was over, Suzanne thanked the newscaster for coming and for bringing Brianne the gift. After the reporter had left the room, Brianne told her mother she liked how the girl had to learn to be a ballerina. "But Mom," she said, "I just want to learn to walk."

Brianne Kiner, with the aid of her physical therapist,
learning to walk on her own again.

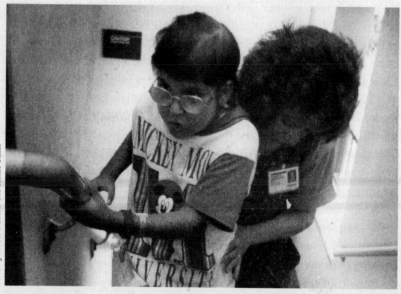

Photo by Teresa Tamura/The Seattle Times

The rehab went on for weeks. One morning the therapist told Brianne she was ready to try walking on her own. She helped Brianne to her feet and then put a walking cane in Brianne's right hand. Her balance shaky, Brianne rested her weight on the cane as the therapist stood at her left side, her arm around Brianne's waist for support. Then, using the cane, Brianne took five baby steps across the wooden floor of the therapy room. The soles of her shoes scuffed the floor. Otherwise, the room was silent.

After the fifth step, Brianne stopped and let go of the cane. Her right arm fell limp to her side. The therapist took a firm hold of her waist but did not hold her up. On her own, Brianne resumed walking. Her knees barely bent. Splints ran from her ankles to her knees. Yet she plodded forward, taking short, determined steps. Then her right foot slipped backward, causing her to stumble.

The therapist paused, allowing Brianne to regain her balance. The right leg moved forward again. Brianne kept going, walking right out the door and into the hallway. The hair on the back of her head still hadn't grown back. Her legs were still too skinny. Her skin still had a bronze tone. But she was a thing of beauty. She proved she could walk. The therapist threw her arms around Brianne and Brianne rested her chin on her shoulder. "I just wanted to walk again," she said.

June 29 was a great day. A couple of weeks earlier Brianne had undergone her final surgery, a procedure to reconnect her small intestine. She had recovered and had been deemed fit to go home. The Kiners were all smiles. The hospital staff and the media were on hand to witness the moment. Suzanne and Rex beamed. Brianne was a walking miracle. Without a wheelchair or a cane, she made her way through the hospital corridors to the outdoors, a place she hadn't been in almost six months.

Wearing a suit and tie for the occasion, Rex removed his jacket and gave it to Brianne. She put it on over her blue hospital gown. The coat dwarfed her, reaching well beneath her knees and making her arms look like those of a scarecrow. Everyone laughed. Brianne was going home.

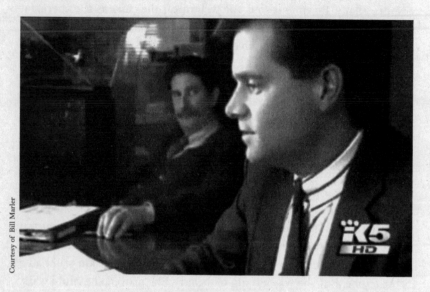

*Bill Marler was turned down when he asked Keller Rohrback
to make him a partner.*

28

JUST AN ASSOCIATE

Wednesday, August 11, 1993

BILL WAS STARTING TO GET ANXIOUS. IT HAD BEEN ROUGHLY THREE months since his initial contact with the Kiner family. He'd had countless meetings and conversations with Suzanne since then. He had negotiated to have Jack in the Box pay for Brianne's rehabilitation treatment and in-home nursing care. He had helped hire a case manager to coordinate Brianne's treatment. And he had done the same with health care professionals to administer medication and conduct therapy—all on Piper's nickel. Bill had even helped the family with media and publicity.

But he still didn't have a retainer agreement authorizing him to act in their behalf. Lynn Sarko was a stickler for tight conformity to bar rules—and to make sure the firm got paid. The firm had put its foot down and crafted a comprehensive retainer agreement for the Kiner family to sign. It specifically made clear that no other lawyers would advise or represent the family. That included Suzanne's brother, Garry, who had continued to try to manage Suzanne's legal affairs from a distance.

On a Saturday afternoon, Bill packed Morgan into the car seat and drove out to Port Townsend to meet Suzanne and Brianne for an outdoor concert where Suzanne's eldest daughter was performing. As they sat on a blanket together, Bill noticed that Brianne's hair had started to grow back, and the natural color of her skin tone was returning. But she still had virtually no mobility. In some ways, she was a lot like one-year-old Morgan—smiling and still.

When it was over, Bill pulled the retainer from his pocket. Before handing it to Suzanne, he looked her in the eye. "What involvement do you want your brother to have in the case?"

"My brother is not my lawyer. My brother is my brother. You're my lawyer."

Bill handed her the retainer agreement. The language specified that her brother would have no further role in representing her. The strict legal language felt harsh to Suzanne. But she understood. She signed the agreement and handed it back to Bill.

That night, Bill took Julie and Morgan out for dinner. They had reason to celebrate. In addition to all the clients that were part of Keller Rohrback's massive class-action suit against Jack in the Box, Bill had signed up more than a dozen clients whose children had suffered severe injuries from HUS. And now the Kiners were signed up, too.

"These cases are going to be lucrative for the firm," Bill told Julie. "It's good for business. And it's something that I brought in on my own."

He was finally getting to the point where he'd hoped he'd end up when he had joined Keller Rohrback nearly four years earlier. He was building up an impressive stable of personal-injury clients.

"I think these guys need to make me a partner," Bill said.

Julie agreed.

"But I'm not sure they're going to do it," he told her.

"Why wouldn't they?"

"Well, you have to be at the firm for seven years before you're eligible for partner. But given the trajectory of my practice, I think they should think outside the box."

He decided the time had come to discuss his status at the firm with Sarko.

On four separate occasions, Lynn Sarko had backed his car into the same post in the parking garage beneath Keller Rohrback's law offices. He wasn't a bad driver, just a distracted one. Each time he hit the post he was simultaneously lighting a cigar while backing up.

Doing two things at once was characteristic of a guy who was too busy to slow down. He was up to almost five hundred clients in the class-action litigation against Exxon, primarily fishermen and cannery workers that had been displaced by the *Exxon Valdez* oil spill. By deciding to try the case himself, Sarko was inundated with pretrial preparation. Plus he was going to have to relocate to Alaska for about a year. At the same time, he was pressing ahead full steam on the antitrust lawsuits on behalf of nuclear and conventionally fueled power plants that had fallen victim to a price-fixing scheme at the hands of steel suppliers and installers. Those cases were coming up for trial, too. On top of all this, he still had to manage the firm, which was akin to running a company.

All of this was weighing on him when Bill entered his office with a skip in his step. His mind elsewhere, Sarko hardly acknowledged Bill's presence.

Bill brought up the Kiners and the fact that they'd signed the retainer. Expecting praise, Bill got none. Instead, Sarko's reaction felt more like "It's about time."

"I think this case is going to make the firm a lot of money," Bill said confidently.

Preoccupied, Sarko mumbled something. While he certainly valued Kiner, to Sarko "a lot of money" was what the Exxon case was going to bring. In the big scheme of things, the firm stood to earn a lot more off an oil spill than from a food poisoning outbreak.

"I think you need to make me a partner," Bill continued.

Finally, Sarko looked up. His patience was wearing thin when it came to Bill's disregard for protocols and his unfamiliarity with the way a large law firm was run. Among other things, the firm had a policy that required associates to spend seven years at the firm before being eligible for partner. Bill had yet to hit the four-year mark. That alone made it an easy call for Sarko.

"Bill, we're just not going to do that," he said dismissively.

The conversation didn't last five minutes.

Deflated, Bill trudged back to his office and shut the door.

Sarko felt Bill had a lot of nerve seeking partnership status just for signing Kiner as a client. "At the firm you get credit for *winning* a case, not *beginning* a case," he explained. "So it seems petulant . . . coming in and saying he wants to be a partner 'because I have a new case.' Show me the judgment or the dismissal. You get credit for winning the race, not showing up at the starting line."

Bill saw a double standard. It seemed convenient for Sarko to take a hard-line stance on the seven-year rule now that he was managing partner. Never mind that the firm had elevated Sarko to partner status after just two years at the firm as an associate.

There were other disparities at the firm. Partners would reap a percentage of the fees in all the big HUS cases that Bill had brought into the firm. But as an associate, Bill would not. He'd get only his base salary. Normally, none of this stuff mattered to Bill. In the back of his mind he kept telling himself that his time would come. But lately he wasn't so sure. It seemed that no matter how hard he worked at Keller Rohrback, he couldn't get noticed. And apparently, reeling in the most celebrated personal-injury case in the city wasn't going to change his fortunes either. The firm seemed perfectly content to continue paying him fifty thousand dollars a year and just to say thanks when the *Jack in the Box* case came to an end.

Feeling underappreciated, Bill walked down to Pinkney Rohrback's office in search of advice. The firm bore his name and he'd been a partner there for forty-three years. A former president of the Seattle–King County Bar Association, Rohrback was far and away the most distinguished member of the firm. He knew all the luminaries in Seattle's legal circles, and the luminaries all knew and respected him.

At sixty-nine, Rohrback still showed up for work every day. His intellect and wit remained sharp as a tack. But his body could no longer keep pace with his mind. His clothes no longer fit. The suits he'd been wearing for the past twenty years were now baggy and long, and the bottoms of his pants legs were frayed from shuffling his feet when he walked. Only a few stray gray hairs poked from his bald head.

Bill peeked in Rohrback's office and found him hunched over his old metal desk. "Pink, can I talk to you?"

Looking up, Pinkney waved Bill in without saying a word.

Bill couldn't help noticing the scarce furnishings—metal, squeaky, and cold. There was no artwork on the walls either, just a few poorly framed, faded family pictures. It was a stark contrast from Sarko's office.

"What's on your mind?" Rohrback asked.

Bill told him about signing up the Kiners, and he shared his views on where he thought the case was headed. Then he revealed the rift with Sarko.

Rohrback didn't say much.

Bill explained that he felt Sarko and others were trying to push him out of the way even though he was the one with all the client contact. Then Bill told him he was contemplating something he thought he'd never do—leaving Keller Rohrback. "What should I do?" Bill asked.

Rohrback maintained a stoic expression. He was the keeper of many secrets, including one about himself. His doctor had recently informed him that he was dying of cancer. He had little time left. Sarko was the only person at the firm who knew any of this, and he knew only because Rohrback figured the managing partner deserved a heads-up from the founding partner. As Rohrback thought about Bill's question, he didn't disclose his medical situation. But it couldn't help coloring his answer.

"Bill, you always have to do the right thing for your client and the right thing for your family," Rohrback advised, expressionless. "And everything else will work out fine."

Earlier in his career, Rohrback undoubtedly would have treated the feud between Sarko and Bill more seriously. But a man facing death has a different perspective on the day-to-day stuff. It's all pretty trivial to him.

Rohrback asked Bill about Julie and Morgan. Like everyone else, he had a soft spot for Julie.

Then Bill stood up to leave. "Thanks, Pink," he said.

Pinckney nodded and returned to what he was doing.

Bill couldn't help searching for a nugget of wisdom in Pinckney's simple advice. "Do right by your client and your family" seemed cliché. But Bill noted the order—client and then family. Rohrback was all about order and priority. Yet Bill didn't think Pinckney placed his job over his family. Rather, it seemed that what Pinckney was saying was that if a lawyer did right by his client, he did right by his family. In other words, he was the same man and saw the world the same way, whether in the role of a lawyer or of a father and husband.

It had been a long day filled with disappointment. Bill left the office with a colleague and headed for the ferry. They frequently commuted together and even had reserved parking spaces side by side at a parking lot near the ferry terminal on Bainbridge Island. When they reached their vehicles, Bill popped the hood on his 1963 pickup and retrieved a quart of transmission fluid from behind the driver's seat. The transmission leaked so much fluid that there were spots all over the ground where he parked. At least two or three times a week he had to add fluid.

"You really need to get a new car," his colleague said, watching Bill try to reach across the engine without getting grease on his suit. "This is becoming a Superfund site."

The guy laughed at his own joke as he climbed into his brand-new sports car and sped off. Bill figured the guy would really laugh if he saw where Bill lived. Shortly after joining the firm, he and Julie bought a tiny cabin on the edge of an Indian reservation just off Bainbridge Island. The place had no insulation and no heating system other than a small fireplace. The electric wiring and the plumbing were outdated. The roof leaked. And the floor was rotted out. Even the shower—a tin box—needed replacing. Unable to afford contractors, Bill and Julie set about fixing the place up on their own, along with a little help from Bill's father and a neighbor who possessed rudimentary carpentry skills.

Little by little they made the place comfortable. But when Julie gave birth to Morgan in April 1992, things got really tight in the five-hundred-square-foot home. Their daughter slept in a crib in the laundry room. Her changing table was the top of the washer and dryer. It was getting harder and harder not to notice that the lawyers Bill worked alongside lived in spacious homes, drove expensive cars, and took vacations outside the U.S. Bill and Julie didn't even own passports.

As soon Bill got home, Julie asked how it had gone with Sarko.

"It was a very short meeting. Basically, there's no way he'd consider me for partner."

Julie frowned.

"It was a 'You're beneath me' kind of thing," Bill continued. "He didn't say that. But it felt like 'How dare you?' I probably should have taken him out to dinner and kissed his ring."

"So it was no partnership, no bonus, no nothing?" she asked.

"Sarko intends to keep me in my place. They're going to keep paying me fifty thousand dollars a year and when the case is over, it's over."

"It doesn't seem fair," she said.

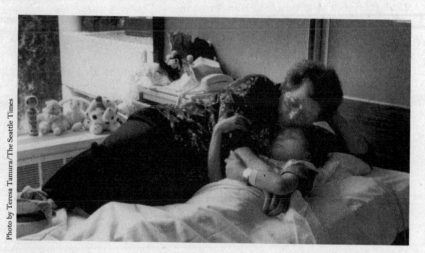

Suzanne Kiner stayed at Brianne's side through every step of rehabilitation. This picture was taken at Children's Hospital in Seattle.

29

IT'S PERSONAL

FOODBORNE DISEASE DOESN'T JUST TEAR UP INTESTINES AND RAVAGE the kidneys of children. It beats the hell out of parents in emotional ways, wears down marital relations, and turns functional families into dysfunctional ones. The Kiners experienced all of this after Brianne left the hospital. Instantly, they discovered their house was no longer a home. Nurses, therapists, and doctors were constantly there. There were ongoing and unanticipated medical problems to address. Brianne had developed diabetes and asthma as a result of the *E. coli* poisoning. Every day began with a regimen of finger pricks and medications, all of which had to be carefully documented. There were more medications at midday, and an insulin injection before dinner and a finger stick and more pills afterward.

For Suzanne and Rex, it felt like a never-ending onslaught. They had no privacy, no time to rest, and no opportunity to replenish their relationship. It got to a point where it seemed as if all they did was argue. At the same time, the couple grappled with something that all parents of food poisoning victims struggle with: guilt.

"I'm the guy who took Bri to Jack in the Box," Rex recalled. "With my background, we should have stayed with the practice of 'One hamburger, one cow.'" It was Rex's way of saying that he never should have taken Brianne to a fast-food chain for a hamburger. It was brutally unfair to hold himself responsible. But it's the kind of thing parents do.

It got to a point where Rex and Suzanne separated. Neither of them wanted to argue anymore. After Rex moved out, the in-home nurses and Brianne's medical case manager began having serious concerns for Suzanne's emotional health. She was diagnosed with post-traumatic stress syndrome and after bravely weathering months of hospitalization and rehab with Brianne, Suzanne was really struggling.

Bill started getting firsthand reports.

The more he heard, the more Bill feared this would all come to a head. But he wasn't sure what to do about it. In his short legal career, he had never encountered this sort of situation with a client.

At the same time, he had his own personal problems to work out. The situation at Keller Rohrback was gnawing at him. Answering to a master was really starting to rub him the wrong way. And to him, Sarko felt like a master. Maybe all the other lawyers at the firm didn't mind Sarko's brand of leadership. Bill was wired differently. His contribution to the *E. coli* litigation seemed utterly beside the point. It was time for another talk with Julie.

"You know, honey," Bill said, "I think I should leave the firm and go somewhere where I can continue to work on the *Kiner* case and these other *E. coli* cases the way I want."

That, of course, implied that Bill's clients would follow him if he left the firm. He and Julie weighed the pros and cons.

The case for staying was straightforward. After bouncing around from firm to firm, Bill finally had a steady salary. That was a big deal now that they had a mortgage and a baby, especially since Julie had left the workforce to be a stay-at-home mom. If Bill walked away from the firm, they might not be able to afford their house payments. Another reason for staying was that Bill liked his colleagues, and Keller Rohrback was a nice place to work.

The case for leaving was even simpler: one, Bill was fighting with the managing partner; two, Bill would *always* fight with the managing partner; and three, the managing partner would always win.

But there was more to it. The *Kiner* case had become Bill's baby. He had an emotional investment in the outcome, and he viewed Brianne's injuries more through the eyes of a parent than a lawyer. "I've seen her with her whole body open," he told Julie. "No one else at the firm has ever even met Brianne. To them, the Kiners are a dollar sign."

And now that Brianne's case was about to take on a high-profile political tone, Bill was eager to push that agenda, but Keller Rohrback was not as gung ho for political activism.

Julie was convinced that Bill would never be happy staying at Keller Rohrback.

If a good opportunity to go elsewhere came along, Bill decided he'd take it.

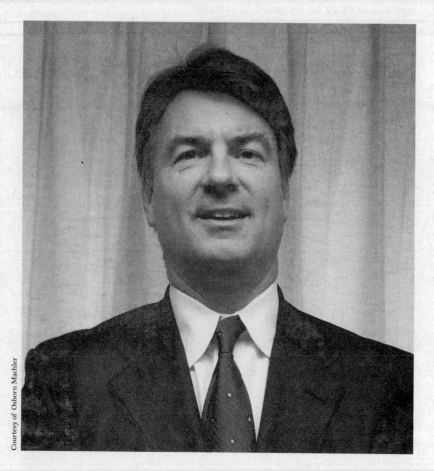

Seattle attorney Simeon Osborn bumped into Bill Marler on a Seattle street at a time when Marler was contemplating changing law firms.

30

LUCKY

Simeon "Sim" Osborn was tall and muscular and had broad shoulders and a Broadway smile. He had played college football before going on to law school. Even though he wore an expensive business suit, it was easy to picture him with a football tucked under his arm, crashing into the end zone, kicking up turf with his cleats as cheerleaders shook their pom-poms. He became a lawyer who preferred not to try cases. Deal making was more Osborn's style.

Osborn's greatest asset as a lawyer was his salesmanship acumen and his connections. His ability to consistently generate more and more clients for his law firm was very valuable. In the competitive world of tort law, firms love a guy who brings business through the doors. And no one did that better than Sim Osborn. He insisted that he could make money without an office; all he needed was a car and a telephone booth. He just seemed to know everybody.

One afternoon Osborn stepped out of his office and headed up the street to get a bite for lunch. Bill was coming down the street in the opposite direction. The two of them had known each other casually for a few years. It had been about a week since Bill had made up his mind to leave Keller Rohrback, but he hadn't come up with a place to go.

"Hey, Sim, how are you?" Bill said.

"B-i-i-i-i-ll," Osborn said, flashing his trademark wide grin.

Minutes later they were seated at a counter, discussing their careers over slices of pizza. The conversation quickly gravitated to Jack in the

Box and Brianne Kiner. It didn't take long for Bill's situation at Keller Rohrback to surface.

Osborn didn't hesitate. "Why don't you come to my firm?" he said.

Bill was instantly intrigued. Osborn's partner was George Kargianis, the highly respected trial lawyer who had arbitrated the previous case in which Bill had faced off against Piper. Kargianis was a bit of a trailblazer. He had been the first lawyer in Washington to file a lawsuit against the tampon industry alleging toxic shock syndrome. He had also brought the first litigation involving the Dalkon Shield, an intrauterine contraceptive device. Through these cases, he had made a name for himself—not to mention a great deal of money—in the area of personal-injury law.

Osborn explained that he and Kargianis were making some internal changes to their practice, including adding another partner, a guy by the name of Mike Watkins, a former prosecutor now in private practice. Bill would make a great fit, too.

Bill couldn't help being interested. It was hard not to be impressed by Osborn, with his *GQ* looks, a shiny new black Porsche, Italian suits, and a pretty blond wife who was a news anchor for one of the network affiliates in Seattle. The guy just seemed to be firing on all cylinders. Working with guys like him and Kargianis could be ideal. Bill and Osborn agreed to keep talking.

Early September 1993

Suzanne called Bill with some exciting news. In the wake of the outbreak, a group of parents and consumers had formed an advocacy group called Safe Tables Our Priority (STOP), dedicated to making America's food system safer and more transparent. In an attempt to get new legislation passed, STOP had organized a foodborne illness symposium on Capitol Hill set for September 21. Ohio senator Howard Metzenbaum had agreed to co-sponsor the event and a large number of lawmakers and food safety regulators were expected to be in attendance. Best of all, STOP had asked Suzanne and Brianne to travel to DC and testify at the symposium.

A big proponent of striking while the iron is hot, Bill encouraged Suzanne to go. Vice President Al Gore had just come out with a statement saying that responsibility for meat inspections should be transferred from the USDA to the FDA. Metzenbaum was floating the idea of giving inspection authority to the Consumer Product Safety Commission. Bill had his doubts that either of these changes would solve the problem. But he liked the fact that the spotlight was squarely on the USDA, and political pressure was mounting to make changes to the way food safety was regulated. By going to the symposium, Brianne and Suzanne would only add to the momentum.

Bill immediately started thinking about how to maximize the opportunity. There was no need to spend time crafting a speech for Suzanne and Brianne. Their experience spoke for itself. Instead, Bill had his mind on how to make the experience more visual to the lawmakers who would be at the symposium, something to really drive home just how destructive *E. coli* could be. To change the politics of food, the problem had to be personalized. The graphic photographs Mike Canaan had taken of Brianne were a good place to start. But Bill had something a little grander in mind—a professionally produced video of Brianne and her illness.

With Suzanne's permission, Bill placed a call to one of the top television news anchors in Seattle and asked her to produce a short thirty-minute film that showed just how much Brianne and her family had suffered as a result of eating bad meat. The news anchor agreed to begin working on the project right away.

September 21, 1993
Washington, DC

Roni Austin had heard all the talk and read all the stories about Brianne Kiner's miraculous recovery. When Roni was invited to testify at a symposium alongside Brianne and Suzanne, she hesitated. She definitely wanted to participate—that was Roni's way of helping bring changes to the meat-safety laws. She owed that to Lauren. But participating was going to mean coming face-to-face with the Kiners, and Roni wasn't sure she could handle that. Suzanne had defied the doctors and conventional wisdom by refusing to remove her daughter from life support, and her daughter had survived. For Roni, it was impossible not to second-guess her own decision to remove Lauren from life support, even though doctors assured her that Lauren had suffered irreversible brain damage as a result of the complications brought on by the *E. coli* poisoning. Still, the loss was something Roni had to live with every day.

On the flight to DC from San Diego, Roni choked back tears, unable to stop wondering, *What is Brianne going to be like?*

The night before the symposium, all the parents who planned to testify gathered at the restaurant in the brownstone hotel where they were all staying. The anticipation of meeting Brianne had Roni in knots.

Brianne entered the restaurant. She was wearing glasses, a Mickey Mouse sweatshirt, and tennis shoes. Other than being a little slow-footed, Brianne looked like a typical ten-year-old girl. Roni was horrified. *This could be Lauren*, she thought.

Tortured by the would-have, could-have, should-have questions, Roni was unsure she'd be able to deliver her testimony. The guilt was eating her up inside. At the same time, Roni couldn't help feeling resentment toward Suzanne. *At least Suzanne has her daughter*, she thought to herself. It was hard not to think that way.

But then Roni found herself standing just a few feet from Brianne. Instinctively, Roni put her arms around her and squeezed, and the embrace did something to her. In Roni's mind, Brianne suddenly represented Lauren.

Looking on, Suzanne felt guilty, too. *E. coli* had killed Roni's daughter. The handful of other mothers on hand for the symposium had also lost a child to foodborne illness. In a strange way, Suzanne felt unworthy of being there because her child had survived. It was awful.

When Roni and Suzanne started talking, the tension evaporated, and tears flowed . . . tears borne of guilt, grief, and agony. There was some anger behind those tears, too. Anger directed at the food industry and the regulators and lawmakers that had shirked their responsibilities. By the following morning, Suzanne and Roni were ready to vent their frustration at the symposium.

Suzanne addressed the distinguished panel, the top of a Diet Pepsi bottle poking out from the baggy pocket of her oversized dress. With no prepared remarks and without notes, she spoke with raw emotion. Her blow-by-blow account of Brianne's experience brought some attendees to tears. When one of the hearing organizers began holding up a cue card indicating Suzanne had exceeded her five-minute limit, Suzanne kept on talking. She wanted to make sure to get her points across to the representatives on hand from the Department of Agriculture. "The USDA is directly responsible," she said, pointing to her daughter's injuries.

Roni Austin was shocked that such a stirring speech could come from a woman who looked so disheveled. But there was something majestic about a shoeless mother speaking truth to power on behalf of her daughter.

After Suzanne finished, the panel saw a clip from the video that Bill had produced back in Seattle. It changed the tone of the hearing. It was hard to watch, but at the same time it was impossible to look away. Then Brianne spoke briefly. "All this happened," she said softly, "because I asked my mother for a hamburger."*

By the time Roni took her place on the dais two seats down from New Jersey congressman Robert Torricelli, her stomach was in knots. She'd never done anything like this. With a blown-up portrait of Lauren and her puppy propped up on an easel behind her, Roni began by telling the audience about the day Lauren dropped to her knees with stomach cramps at their home. She finished by telling the audience that Lauren was buried in her Christmas dress a week later. "This is not okay," Roni said, her voice giving way to tears. "This is not okay."

After it was over, Suzanne called Bill from DC with a rundown on what had transpired at the symposium. She had been interviewed by members of the Washington press corps, and STOP had informed Suzanne that it was pushing for congressional hearings later in the fall, and the group wanted Suzanne to come back and testify again.

Bill was thrilled at her news. Listening, it was all he could do to keep from telling her his, that he was changing law firms. But he held his tongue. Besides, he still had to close the loop with Sim Osborn and George Kargianis.

They'd had a series of follow-up telephone conversations, and it was clear to Bill that they wanted him. A face-to-face meeting had been scheduled to discuss the details of what a new partnership would look like.

---

*Brianne asked her mother for a hamburger, but her father is the one who took her to Jack in the Box.

Bill figured it was time to give Julie the good news. He told her he was pretty sure he'd found a new law firm that was willing to make him a partner.

Julie sensed some hesitation on Bill's part.

"If I leave Keller Rohrback," Bill said, "this could be devastating for us financially because they might come after us." Bill explained that he was certain Suzanne and Brianne Kiner would follow him, along with other clients, and that would anger the firm. It might go as far as to sue him over the loss of clients.

"But the alternative isn't good either, Bill," Julie said. "You can't continue working for Sarko."

Bill agreed. "I'm going to have to hire an attorney to figure out how to do this."

31

FIDUCIARY MATTERS

BILL CONSULTED INFORMALLY WITH TWO LAWYERS ABOUT THE BEST way to leave one firm and join another. Looking at Bill's situation, both attorneys said the same thing: Before walking out the door, Bill should line up the clients—especially Brianne Kiner—to follow him. Then he should walk away and not look back. Lawyers refer to this as the Pearl Harbor approach.

The advice didn't sit well with Bill. That wasn't the way he wanted to leave. Besides, there were other factors to consider. A lot of effort went into setting up a class-action suit that now included close to two hundred clients. Bill didn't want to disrupt that. However, he did hope *Kiner* and the other individual HUS cases he was handling on an individual basis would follow him. But with so much national publicity swirling around the outbreak, he didn't want to create a sideshow with his departure. This had to be handled properly. It was clear he needed a more sophisticated approach.

He turned to the best lawyer he knew when it came to dealing with trouble: Brad Keller, one of the founding partners at Byrnes & Keller, considered some of the toughest, hardest-charging trial lawyers in Seattle. Though highly respected in legal circles, the firm wasn't well liked by the public. That was because their clients wore black hats—a mining company accused of securities fraud, a tobacco company facing consumer-protection and antitrust charges, *Fortune* 500 companies in contract disputes over hundreds of millions of dollars, and national law firms facing civil or criminal charges for malfeasance. Byrnes & Keller liked these clients because they had deep pockets. And these clients like Byrnes & Keller because they won.

Bill's first job out of law school was as an associate assigned to Brad Keller. Byrnes & Keller had a policy against hiring anyone with less than four years of trial experience, but Bill had talked his way into a job by convincing Keller that he was worth an exception and promising to go quietly if the firm wasn't satisfied with his performance. Nine

Attorney Brad Keller represented Bill Marler when he decided to leave his old law firm and join a new one.

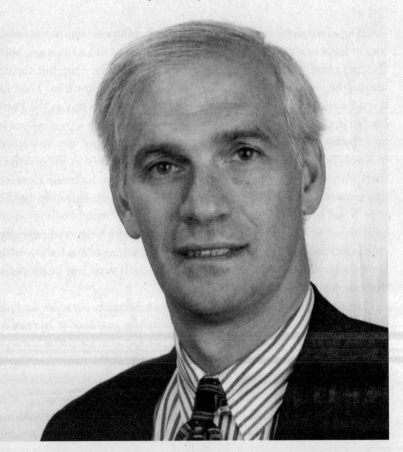

months later Keller called Bill into his office to inform him he was being let go. He simply lacked the kind of experience the firm needed in its associates. It was a humiliating start to Bill's law career. But during those nine months that Bill worked alongside Keller, he had watched him deftly navigate business clients through some harrowing situations where careers, reputations, and fortunes were on the line. Keller had also represented numerous, well-known Seattle attorneys through difficult disputes involving ethics and professional responsibility.

Bill decided to call him.

Keller was pleasantly surprised to hear from Bill. They hadn't talked since Keller let him go. Impressed that Bill held no grudge, Keller asked how he could help.

Bill explained his situation.

With all the press coverage devoted to Brianne Kiner and her remarkable recovery, Keller understood the predicament right away. If Bill switched firms after landing the most prized personal-injury client in the city, there would surely be hell to pay.

Bill told him what a couple of other lawyers had advised.

"That sounds very aggressive and unnecessarily exposing you to personal risk," Keller said.

Risk wasn't what Bill needed. The thought of a nasty fight with Keller Rohrback made him ill. Between Jack in the Box and their insurance companies and their lawyers, Bill was fighting on enough fronts.

Keller agreed.

"Look, I'm not going to stay at this law firm," Bill told Keller. "But at the end of the day, how do I do this in a way that is best for the client and is ethically appropriate, so I don't end up in a squabble with Keller Rohrback?"

Keller had been down this road with other lawyers, many of them far more established in their careers than Bill. And they typically asked: "How can I get what's good for me and protect myself?" Bill's question put the client's interest ahead of his own. This told Keller something— he wasn't looking across the desk at the same lawyer that he'd let go a few years earlier for lack of experience. Rather, Bill was displaying the kind of wisdom Keller rarely saw in senior partners. He agreed to represent him.

But he wasn't prepared to just spout off advice. Lawyers tend to look at cases simply as *matters*, but Keller could see this case was much more than a legal matter to Bill. He was personally and emotionally invested in the Kiner family's tragedy on a level that went far beyond serving them professionally as a lawyer. It felt more like a mission. It was pretty clear that Bill felt a personal obligation to the Kiners and the other families whose children had HUS. With that in mind, Keller felt a special obligation to Bill. He asked for some time to research a few issues and promised to get back to him as soon as he had answers.

Denis Stearns had been playing a game of cat and mouse with Bill over discovery documents, rejecting his broad requests for all documents pertaining to "meat," but he was losing ground. Bill kept at it.

Stearns refused on grounds that Bill hadn't been specific enough in his demand. *Meat* is a very broad term. On the Jack in the Box menu, it could be beef patties, hot dogs, ham on breakfast sandwiches, chicken, and numerous other items.

This case is about E. coli, Stearns decided. *For purposes of answering the discovery requests, what's relevant to this case is ground beef products.*

He sent Bill a letter limiting his request. "For purposes of our response, we are producing all documents having to do with any ground beef related sandwich." He also sent Bill a menu showing all the other meat products that contain no ground beef.

Pleased that he'd been getting the better of Bill in this contest of precision, Stearns got nervous when he saw the latest decision issued by the Washington State Supreme Court published toward the end of September. In it the court reprimanded a pharmaceutical company and its defense attorneys for abusing the discovery process. The abuse had to do with failing to produce all the internal documents that plaintiffs were entitled to see. The Supreme Court outlined a new standard. When deciding not to produce documents, defense lawyers had to make clear what was being withheld.

Ever the stickler for rules and regulations, Stearns saw this as a big red flag. He had been careful not to mislead Bill on what he was and wasn't turning over. But Stearns wasn't as confident that the in-house lawyers for Jack in the Box had been as careful. And ultimately, they were the ones that had access to the records. Each time a documents request came in from Bill, Stearns would narrow it before forwarding it on to the Jack in the Box headquarters, where a corporate lawyer would respond by pulling documents that complied with the request.

But what if Jack in the Box's in-house counsel had not been as exhaustive as he should have been? What if there were documents in the files that Bill was entitled to see? Uneasy, Stearns shared his concerns with Piper, who had the same fear.

"We really need to go down there," Stearns told Piper. "We need to look at all their documents. I want to physically go through their file cabinets."

Piper didn't need to be convinced. He loved the idea of dispatching Stearns to San Diego for other reasons. It would generate lots more billable hours and broaden Piper's already expansive domain over the case, two things he adored. He agreed to call Jack in the Box and inform them that Stearns would be coming down to go through all their internal records.

The more he looked into Bill's legal options, the more it became clear to Brad Keller that Bill's decision to leave Keller Rohrback was fraught with risk whether or not the clients followed him. If Kiner and the other *E. coli* victims chose to remain with Keller Rohrback, Bill would have walked away from the biggest case of his career and the most secure job he'd ever had. He'd second-guess that decision for the rest of his life. The more likely scenario, however, was that the clients *would* go with him. That presented an even greater set of challenges. For starters, the *E. coli* cases were incredibly labor-intensive. By joining a much smaller firm with only three colleagues, all of whom had their own caseload, Bill would basically be taking on a workload that was currently being shouldered by a half dozen partners and a stable of paralegals and secretaries between Keller Rohrback and Chris Pence's firm. The *Kiner* case alone could drown Bill.

But that wasn't all. On top of a colossal workload, he'd have a fight on his hands with his former partners. There simply was no way around it. There was no way lawyers would let him go quietly while so much revenue walked out the door. That meant Bill would be fighting Jack in the Box on one front and his old law firm on another front.

Over lunch, Keller spelled out Bill's options.

First, although Bill had personally signed up Kiner and many other clients who were victims of *E. coli*, those clients technically belong to the firm. Associates were employees and any work they generated was the property of the employer.

Second, Bill owed fiduciary responsibilities to his firm. One of those responsibilities prevented him from using his relationship with a client to the disadvantage of the firm.

Third, clients had an absolute right to decide whom they wanted to represent them, whether it was the firm or an individual attorney.

"So," Keller said, "how do you let the client exercise their right to decide who they want as their lawyer, while fulfilling your duty of loyalty to the law firm?"

"Yeah, how do I do that?"

"The only way to do it is to really try and create a level opportunity for the lawyer on one hand and the law firm on the other."

That didn't mean Bill couldn't have *any* discussion with the Kiners and the others. Giving the clients a simple heads-up about his intention to change firms was permissible. The professional responsibility guidelines allowed for a lawyer to let a client know that he was potentially going to explore other employment opportunities. "What you can't do is actively solicit them and line them up and wire it," Keller said. "Because then you're doing it while you're in the employment of the firm, and you're wresting the clients away from the firm."

It all boiled down to the fact that an individual lawyer couldn't use his relationship with a client to the disadvantage of the firm. Bill could see how this approach might give Keller Rohrback a leg up in holding onto the clients. But he decided to play it safe, going as far as to avoid giving the Kiners and the others a heads-up.

But what about the contents of the case files? The *Kiner* file and some of the other more serious cases were in his office. The files were filled with information Bill had compiled, along with important contact and personal information on the clients. A couple of lawyers had told Bill that he should photocopy the files before leaving the firm. Bill asked Keller's opinion.

"If you're going to do the Pearl Harbor approach," Keller said, "that's what you do on the way out the door."

But Keller advised strongly against it. "The file belongs to the client," Keller said. "In order to take a client's file with you, you must first have the client's consent. And you can't get that consent without wiring it with the client."

He suggested a more conservative approach: to write a letter to each of the clients *after* leaving Keller Rohrback, to inform them of Bill's decision to change firms and offer them the opportunity to remain with the firm or follow him. For those who chose to stick with Bill, he should then seek the file from Keller Rohrback. "The old firm can copy the file for its records," Keller said. "But it must move the file."

None of this was going to be easy. A lot of work, money, and time had been invested in the *E. coli* cases, both by Bill and his firm. Whichever side lost the clients was going to feel cheated.

Bill understood.

Keller wished him well and told Bill to keep him posted. As Bill walked out, Keller reflected on how far Bill had come. He had been a fish out of water when he had come to work for Byrnes & Keller right out of law school. Financial statements and balance sheets—that stuff of complex business litigation—were not Bill's strong suit. Representing people with failing organs and extreme injuries was where he belonged. The question was whether he'd be able to hold on to his clients.

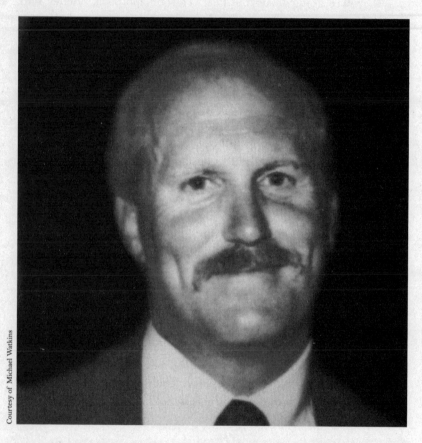

Michael Watkins agreed to join Bill Marler and two other lawyers in the formation of a new law firm called Kargianis, Osborn, Watkins & Marler.

32

YOU HAVE TO TRUST ME

FORTY-FIVE-YEAR-OLD MICHAEL WATKINS HAD BEGUN HIS LAW CAREER in the Orange County district attorney's office. In 1983 he had relocated to Seattle and started up a solo practice doing insurance-defense work. Eventually he had started renting office space from George Kargianis and Simeon Osborn. There had been talk of having Watkins join their firm. The three lawyers had never gotten around to ironing out any details. But now, with Marler in the mix, the time seemed right.

Bill met the three of them at the Sorrento Hotel. Its mahogany furniture, marble-encased fireplaces, and silk-brocade linen and drapery were just the kind of trappings that suited George Kargianis. Known in the legal community as "Gentleman George," he dressed like an aristocrat. He spoke like one, too. His voice could be deep and condescending, his delivery deliberate. But he was ultimately smooth. His friends liked to say he had the kind of touch that could make a silk purse out of a sow's ear.

He took quick command of the gathering, regaling the group with stories before asking Bill a series of questions about his current situation and his aspirations. A pretty good salesman himself, Bill hit it off with Kargianis. It was obvious to each of them that Marler had his hand on the throttle in the *Jack in the Box* case.

"Well you know Bill," Kargianis said in a suave tone, "I like the cut of your jib."

Osborn and Watkins laughed. Bill did, too, despite not being familiar with the expression. All Bill cared about was the fact that Kargianis seemed very eager to start a new law firm: Kargianis, Osborn, Watkins & Marler.

And with the firm's resources, Bill wouldn't have to worry about how to finance the cost of taking on Jack in the Box.

Momentum was building quickly. Osborn had been looking around and had located some new office space overlooking Pike Place Market. He assured the group that the space was among the most exclusive in the city, with exquisite natural wood finishes and picturesque views of Elliott Bay. The lease was ready to sign.

Next the group discussed roles. Kargianis and Osborn were well established with a lengthy list of clients. They'd simply continue doing what they had been doing. Watkins would bring his insurance-defense clients into the firm and his day-to-day responsibilities would remain status quo. Most of the discussion revolved around Bill's role. Everyone agreed that he would spend virtually all his time on *Kiner* and all other *E. coli* cases he was able to reel in. The other lawyers would largely be hands-off. But the firm would provide all the financial resources and office support that Bill needed. And of course, Kargianis was available whenever Bill needed advice from one of the most experienced trial lawyers in the city.

It was all music to Bill's ears. He'd have freedom to manage the cases as he saw fit, financial backing, and partner status. The only thing left to resolve was money. Up front, Bill informed the group that he would not make an attempt to reach out to the nearly two hundred clients in the class-action suit. His new partners felt that was an awful lot of potential business to leave behind, but Bill made it clear that the entire class could be disrupted if some clients opted to leave and others didn't. Instead, he preferred to go after the individual clients that weren't part of the class. The discussion quickly turned to money and how to divide up fees generated by any *E. coli* cases that Bill brought into the office.

They quickly agreed on a simple approach:

- Sixty percent of the fees would go to Bill's three partners, to be dispersed equally among them.

- Forty percent of the fees would go to Bill.

Kargianis, Osborn, and Watkins thought that was more than fair.

The potential windfall from the *Kiner* case was impossible for Bill to downplay. The other lawyers preferred some kind of guarantee that Kiner and the other clients would follow Bill to their firm.

"I can't imagine these people will stay at the firm if I leave," Bill said.

But lawyers like things air tight.

Bill made it clear he would make no efforts whatsoever to contact any of the clients in advance. "You're just going to have to trust me," Bill said.

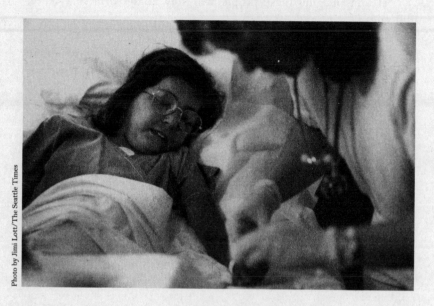

*Brianne Kiner, receiving treatment from a nurse
at Seattle's Children's Hospital.*

33

FOOD-SAFETY ADVOCATES

BILL'S TO DO LIST KEPT GETTING LONGER AND MORE COMPLEX. DENIS Stearns had become like a pesky gnat, constantly coming up with reasons for narrowing Bill's requests for access to Jack in the Box documents. Bill redrafted his interrogatories and sent them back over to Stearns's office.

At the same time, Piper had requested an up-to-date list of all plaintiffs included in the class-action suit. Bill ran through the file and confirmed the number was up to 187. He dashed off a memo to Piper.

Then there was the *Kiner* case. It always seemed to dominate everything on Bill's plate. Every day, it seemed, there was a new twist. Bill wasn't surprised when Congress announced the first in a series of hearings intended to reinvent the federal food-safety system. The goal was to change the way the USDA inspected meat and poultry. Suzanne had been called to testify. Unlike her appearance at the symposium six weeks earlier, this time around she was required to provide a prepared statement in advance. Bill wanted to attend the hearing with her, but he had too many irons in the fire in Seattle. Instead, he went over the draft of her testimony and then sent her off to DC on her own.

Thursday, November 4, 1993
Rayburn House Office Building
Washington, DC

Too determined to be nervous, Suzanne looked on as New York congressman Edolphus Towns called the hearing to order. "The Federal

Government spends $9 billion each year on food-safety activities," Towns said in an angry tone. "But what are taxpayers getting annually for their money? Nine thousand deaths, 80 million people sick, some chronically disabled; eight to seventeen billion dollars in medical costs each year from food tainted with deadly microbes such as *E. coli* O157:H7. If we are truly going to reform health care, we must start with the basics: prevention. We must prevent foodborne disease, not just treat its victims."

Seated at the witness table, Suzanne liked what she was hearing.

"The current federal food-safety system isn't just fragmented; it's broken," Towns continued. "USDA has known for over twenty years that its inspection system cannot detect harmful microbes in meat and poultry, but did absolutely nothing about it."

Then the chairman faced Suzanne. "It is customary," he said, "that all witnesses who appear before this committee are sworn. If you will stand?"

Suzanne stood, raised her right hand, and took the oath.

"Let me say again, we thank you so much for coming," Towns said. "Ms. Kiner."

"My daughter Brianne Kiner laid in a hospital bed for 167 days. For 55 of those days she was dying. Our story begins with a tainted hamburger."

"The most frightening change in Brianne was her mental status. She plummeted from a bright ten-year-old to a frightened two-year-old. Brianne's brain was already beginning to swell. Her voice pitch climbed, and her vocabulary became simpler. My daughter's mind was slipping away, and there was nothing I could do to stop it."

Then came the coma. Suzanne tried to keep her composure. "Her heart was barely functioning. We were asked to plan our daughter's funeral."

She paused and looked into the faces of the members of the panel. "Have you ever planned a child's funeral?" she asked them.

"The recommendation was to pull the plug," Suzanne said. "Ladies and gentlemen, we had a miracle from God. But . . . my daughter lives with an uncertain future."

The next morning, Suzanne telephoned Bill's office from her hotel in DC. She felt good about her testimony.

Bill congratulated her, but he kept the call short. He was too antsy. It was Friday, his last day at the office. None of his colleagues had any idea that it was the last time they'd be seeing Bill Marler around the firm. That was one of the reasons he was so anxious. He couldn't wait to get the day over with.

Just before leaving work at the end of the day, he closed his door and placed a telephone call to Piper.

———————

Seated at his desk, Piper listened as Denis Stearns reported on his research into the Washington State meat-cooking standards.

"The vast majority of the counties in the state were not enforcing the 155-degree standard," Stearns said. "The state test that you take to get a license still listed 140 degrees. Even the inspection report form still said 140 degrees."

In other words, while the state had been quick to publicly pummel Jack in the Box for failing to cook its hamburgers to the new standard, behind the scenes, the state had been very haphazard in enforcing it. At the time of the outbreak, the vast majority of counties in Washington were still working off the 140-degree rule.

Stearns assured Piper that it was worse than that. He had dug up dozens of restaurant-inspection reports done in the weeks prior to the outbreak, where state health inspectors had written things like: "Remember to cook to 140." Even the booklets that counties were handing out to applicants for food-worker permits still said that hamburger had to be cooked to 140 degrees.

"Bottom line," Stearns said, "the new regulation had been passed at the state level but it hadn't filtered down to the local municipalities. It's safe to say that Jack in the Box was by no means the only restaurant not cooking meat to an internal temperature of 155. They're just the only one that got caught."

Piper leaned back in his chair and stretched his suspenders. He did that when he was feeling confident. If the state dared to prosecute Jack in the Box for violating state law, he would embarrass the hell out of state officials by exposing just how derelict the state had been in updating its training manuals and inspection sheets. Shit, county health inspectors weren't even aware of the change. How in the hell could the state expect Jack in the Box to be up to speed? That was the way Piper planned to play it.

Suddenly Piper's phone rang. It was Marler, calling late in the afternoon on a Friday.

"I just want to let you know I'm leaving Keller Rohrback," Bill said.

Piper was stunned. Bill had just sent him the updated list of class-action clients, showing Keller Rohrback was up to nearly two hundred clients. "Damn it, Marler! You're leaving *this*?"

Piper just couldn't get over the idea that Bill would walk away from the biggest case in Seattle.

"After I leave I'm going to let the clients know where I'm going," Bill assured him.

Piper laughed at him for waiting to notify the clients. "Where the hell are you going?" he asked.

"I'm joining George Kargianis's firm."

There was silence on the other end. It took a lot to shock Piper, but this move did. Immediately, Piper relished the possibilities. Piper went way back with Kargianis. Piper's brother had been Kargianis's law school roommate. And Piper and Kargianis had worked together for years.

"Well . . . shit, Marler," Piper said, pleased. "What about the class?"

Bill told him he intended to contact only the Kiners and the clients with HUS. He had no intention of contacting members of the class.

"Why the hell not?" Piper asked.

Bill tried explaining that it would be too much for his firm to take that on. Besides, it would be too disruptive to the clients. Moving a class of nearly two hundred clients would be a lot more complicated than moving a dozen individual cases.

"Oh damn you," Piper said.

It was clear to Bill that all Piper cared about was getting away from Sarko and Pence. He'd much prefer dealing with Bill and Kargianis.

"Bob, I'm not going to make a play for the class," Bill repeated.

Grumpy, Piper told Bill to keep him posted.

34

BREAKING UP IS HARD TO DO

November 7, 1993

No matter how much he fought it, Bill couldn't escape feeling he was about to betray his firm by leaving. It had offered him a position when he desperately needed a job. The firm had been a stable and steady employer. Yet Bill was convinced that the Kiners and the other clients not included in the class-action suit would be better served by him than by Keller Rohrback. Still, it felt an awful lot like a divorce. And relationships are never the same after a divorce. Bill had become more and more restless about how he had chosen to handle his departure. But it wouldn't be the first time he had done something like this.

During the summer between his junior and senior years of high school, Bill had felt really dissatisfied with what he was doing with himself. One Saturday while his parents were off grocery shopping together, he packed a duffle bag and took twenty dollars out of his father's sock drawer. Then he hitchhiked all the way to eastern Washington. Halfway across the state he phoned home and told his parents he was okay, but he wouldn't be home until the fall.

Bill ended up at a gigantic fruit farm, where he got a job as a farmhand alongside migrant farmers of all different ethnic backgrounds. Broke, he started out eating pancake dough or whatever else he could scrounge up, while spending his days moving irrigation lines and picking cherries, apples, and peaches. The living conditions were dank and crude. *Wow,* Bill remembered thinking to himself back then, *I could end up like this if*

I don't apply myself. When he returned home that fall, he buckled down and began thinking seriously about going to law school after college.

Now Bill knew the time had come to leave his comfort zone again. But that didn't make it any easier. "I'm scared to death," Bill told Mike Watkins when they spoke by telephone Sunday afternoon.

Watkins understood. He compared the situation to when a husband sneaks back to his house to retrieve his golf clubs after he's moved out and decided to get a divorce—he shows up when no one's home.

"Listen," Watkins said, "I'll go with you and help you pack up boxes."

It was after nine on Sunday night when Bill and Watkins pulled into the parking garage beneath the Washington Mutual Bank Building. It wasn't hard to find a parking space. When they reached the main lobby it felt deserted. Even the security guard station was unmanned. Their shoes echoed as they walked briskly across the vast marble floor to the bank of elevators leading to the upper floors. Stepping inside, Bill inserted his key card and the elevator began climbing to thirty-second floor. Bill's stomach was in knots. *What if the doors open and someone is standing there?* Keller Rohrback leased the entire thirty-second floor, along with part of the one below it. So the reception desk and waiting area were right off the elevator. *What if someone has come in to work on a Sunday?*

The doors opened and Bill stepped out. The auxiliary lights were on, but that was all. The place was dead quiet. They made a beeline to Bill's office. Once inside, Bill closed the door, dimmed his lights, and turned down the miniblinds on his office window that faced the hallway. Then he started clearing personal items from his desk into a box: family pictures, a letter opener, a paperweight. Watkins went to the bookcase and started packing up Bill's books. As he reached for a set of Continuing Legal Education (CLE) binders, Bill looked up.

"No, no," Bill told him. "That's Keller Rohrback's."

Watkins didn't see the big deal. They were study guides. The firm probably had fifty or a hundred copies. But Bill was adamant.

"I went to the CLE on their nickel," Bill said. "Leave 'em here."

Watkins removed the manuals from the box and put them back on the shelf. Then he grabbed more books.

"No, that's not mine either," Bill said, identifying another book that didn't belong to him. "That has to stay, too."

Watkins took a step back while Bill pointed out the remaining books that should be left behind because they belonged to the firm. They were all manuals and reference books, the sort that the firm probably had dozens and dozens of copies of. It wasn't as if they'd miss this stuff.

Impressed, Watkins said nothing. It was like watching a guy standing on the sidewalk at a deserted intersection at 2:00 a.m., waiting for the Walk sign before he'll step into the crosswalk. He was convinced Bill wouldn't take a paper clip that didn't belong to him.

In less than thirty minutes they were done. Bill's three years at Keller Rohrback were reduced to three boxes. He grabbed two, and Watkins carried the other.

"I've got to go to Pinckney's office," Bill said as he exited his office for the last time. Watkins waited for Bill by the elevators.

In Pinckney's office Bill removed a typed letter from his pocket. He had composed it a few days earlier and had it vetted by Brad Keller. It matter-of-factly stated that he had left the firm and become a partner at Kargianis, Osborn, Watkins & Marler. He placed it on Pinckney's chair and walked out.

The Next Morning

Lynn Sarko had trouble believing what he was seeing. Bill's office was cleaned out . . . empty . . . abandoned. The only explanation was a short note discovered on Pinckney's chair. It indicated Bill had joined another law firm.

Shocked and confused, Sarko checked with other partners to see if any of them knew more. None did. All they could offer was a question: "How could this happen without warning?"

Dumbfounded, Sarko couldn't help wondering if his recent run-in with Bill over talking to the media was behind his exit. "When Bill left," Sarko explained, "that's why I thought he left . . . that there was a fork in the road over me being so upset with him."

Whatever the reason, Sarko was stunned and angry. "I was peeved when Bill left the way he did," Sarko explained. "To have somebody on the team steal out in the middle of the night . . . I chalk it up to youthful indiscretion."

The Jack in the Box litigation was at a critical stage and Bill had a vital role. He was the firm's point man to all the *E. coli*–poisoning victims whose injuries were too severe to be included in the class-action suit. And he was the firm's only line of communication to the Kiner family.

Sarko had one hell of a mess on his hands. He was about to start the trial of his career against Exxon in Alaska. At the same time, the firm had close to two hundred clients in the *Jack in the Box* case, which was advancing rapidly on many fronts. There was a staggering amount of work to do, but Bill's sudden exit had created instant chaos. For one thing, clients had to be contacted and notified that Bill had left and someone else was stepping into his shoes. But who? Bill had controlled the files on those cases and he alone had the personal relationship with these people.

Sarko had another problem—office morale. Lawyers at the firm felt betrayed. So did Sarko, especially since he had defended Bill's maverick moves in the past. "Every time someone in the firm would complain about Bill, I'd support him because I'd see me [as a young lawyer] in it," Sarko explained.

Not this time, however. Bill was now an adversary.

Chris Pence had barely gotten to his office when his phone rang. It was Sarko. He gave Pence the news.

"Wow!" Pence said, unable to grasp it. "That's just shocking."

Sarko agreed.

"What an asshole," Pence said.

Pence took it more personally than many of Bill's colleagues at Keller Rohrback. Bill was the one who had initially suggested Pence join forces with Keller Rohrback. And Pence's best friend, Will Smart, was the one most responsible for Keller Rohrback's having hired Bill. Bill's move felt like betrayal. It hurt—badly. "I was shocked, hurt, and I was outraged," Pence recalled.

Everything about Bill's first day at his new firm was different, starting with the moment he stepped off the ferry in Seattle. Instead of going straight out of the terminal and walking up the hill toward his old office tower, he hung a left and headed up First Avenue toward Pike Place Market until he got to Market Place Tower. He took the elevator to Penthouse Suite A, where his name appeared on a brand-new nameplate over the door to his private office. The woodwork was exquisite. The view was even better. He looked out over Puget Sound.

Seattle solo attorney Chris Pence and Keller Rohrback ended up in a bitter dispute with Marler when he left the firm, and the Kiner family and other clients followed him.

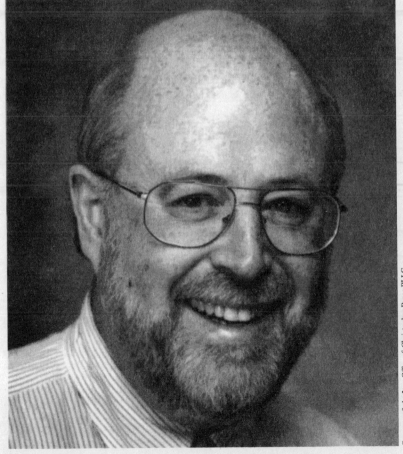

It was hard not to feel he'd arrived. His firm had the penthouse suite. He was a partner now. The other three partners at the firm each drove a Porsche. If materialism was the indication of lawyers' success, Bill had hitched his wagon to the right ones.

His first item of business was to contact the clients he'd worked with at Keller Rohrback. A little over half of them were from the *E. coli* outbreak. The others were people Bill represented on a variety of personal-injury claims. The letters to each of them were already typed, signed, sealed, and mailed before midmorning.

Suzanne Kiner was the first client to contact Bill. She assured him that the family would contact Keller Rohrback and asked to have their file transferred to Bill's new law office immediately. By week's end, Bill had heard from the rest of the *E. coli* victims he had written. All but one had decided to have their cases transferred from Keller Rohrback to him.

Bill placed a call to Piper to update him on the situation.

"What about the class?" Piper asked.

"Bob, I already told you, I'm not making a play for the class," Bill said.

Piper teased him that he didn't have the balls to go after the class, too.

Stearns looked on as Piper got a rundown from Bill on the fallout with Keller Rohrback. Sometimes Stearns felt as if half his billable hours were spent listening to Piper talk on the phone. When the call ended, Piper filled him in on Marler.

Stearns wondered what Piper thought of Marler's move.

"Brash," Piper said. "Brash."

Stearns had his own view. He knew how much Sarko liked deference. Marler definitely didn't show it . . . and never would. Inevitably, Marler had to leave. These were two guys born to lead, not follow.

But Stearns kept all that to himself. Piper didn't need to hear it. He had his own fiefdom to protect.

35

CONTEMPT

THE TIME HAD COME FOR JACK IN THE BOX TO MAKE UP ITS MIND ABOUT what to do with Ken Dunkley. At the management level there were two schools of thought. One was that his carelessness had dealt the company a severe blow and that he should be let go. The other was that Dunkley had been a model, loyal employee and that it was unfair to saddle him with all the blame. Dave Theno was in the second camp.

"Ken was wounded," Theno explained. "I felt sorry for the guy because I knew exactly the position he'd been put in. If I was going to hold one person accountable for allowing the situation to develop that created this outbreak, it wouldn't be Ken. You have to remember that prior to the outbreak, food safety was just a task that had to be part of the drill. At the executive level, the commitment to support food safety as a top priority was very low. This wasn't just Jack in the Box. Everybody was like that."

To some degree, Nugent had come around to Theno's way of thinking. He had concluded that the company's organization chart was flawed. It had to do with who reported to whom. Dunkley was over quality assurance. Food safety fell under quality assurance. Yet Dunkley reported directly to Mo Iqbal, the company's vice president over marketing.

Nugent implemented a series of personnel changes. Dave Theno was promoted to vice president of quality assurance, research and development, and product safety. On the revised organizational chart,

Theno reported directly to Nugent. Finally, Ken Dunkley was moved out of quality assurance altogether and reassigned to work with Iqbal in the marketing division.

Dunkley immediately had his doubts. In the back of his mind he couldn't help thinking that the reason he hadn't been let go was to insure that he remained a friendly witness during the litigation. He also felt he'd been shoved some place he didn't belong. "I had a great deal of pride and satisfaction in R&D for many years," Dunkley explained. "I was widely respected in the industry. But when that stopped and my work changed and I moved out of technical into marketing and restaurant development, I felt a little disconnected from my real passion and my roots—the food part of the business. At the same time, I appreciated that I was still being given opportunity by the company."

However, the new changes fostered resentment on the part of Dunkley toward Theno. "I did feel some animosity toward Dave Theno," Dunkley explained. "He ended up becoming the preeminent food-safety guy and took the spotlight. It was almost symbolic that he ended up heading up the technical area and I ended up in marketing. It wasn't that he pushed or forced me out. But I struggled with that."

It was only a matter of time before this would all come to a head. But Nugent couldn't be bothered with the internal politics. His attention was acutely focused on the company's balance sheet. The outbreak had wreaked havoc on sales. At the same time, the company was spending money hand over fist on public relations and legal fees. Unless revenue picked up, Nugent knew the oldest fast-food chain in the U.S. was doomed. In an attempt to spur sales, he approved deep discounting of the entire menu in all 1,155 restaurants throughout the country. And he hired an ad agency to develop a television ad campaign to win back customers.

It's been said that hell hath no fury like a woman scorned. But a pack of scorned lawyers can be worse. Bill had managed to tick off two law firms, Keller Rohrback and Chris Pence's, and they were bent on a reckoning. Yet the firms had different motivations.

Pence's firm was very small, more like a solo practice. Thanks to his arrangement with Keller Rohrback, he stood to earn a portion of every fee collected from nearly two hundred clients in the class-action suit— a tort lawyer's dream. Plus, he was entitled to a portion of any fees collected from the more severe HUS cases, *Kiner* being the sugar daddy of that group of cases.

Keller Rohrback, on the other hand, was a big, established firm with annual fee revenues that ranged between $20 million and $40 million in any given year. "So the *Kiner* case was important," said Sarko. "But it wasn't financially going to change people's behavior."

Legal fees were certainly on Sarko's mind. But how Bill left and where he ended up were also issues. "It's like a divorce," Sarko explained. "In divorce law the issue is as much about bruised feelings as it is about the economics of it. In law-firm issues it's complicated by the fact that there's a client involved. So it's like a divorce with child custody."

The fact that Bill went to a rival firm added another dimension. "If I leave my spouse, it's one thing," Sarko explained. "If I leave my spouse in the middle of the night and move in with another person, you get a different reaction. People are wondering how long did this go on? Is it really what it is? Is it what it seems? It raises all kinds of ethical issues."

Pence agreed. His first job out of law school had been with the Washington State Bar Council, and subsequently he had done a fair amount of work in the area of legal malpractice. Professional responsibility was an area he knew quite well. He had a suspicion that Bill's departure was the result of very careful planning. The quick landing with Kargianis and the presence of Brad Keller offering advice were key indicators. "It was totally orchestrated," Pence said.

No matter what, one thing was clear: Bill's old firm was gearing up to sue his new one.

36

WIZARDS OF OZ

Mid-December 1993

IN PERSONAL-INJURY CASES INVOLVING MINORS REQUIRING EXTENSIVE, long-term medical care, a life-care planner (LCP) has the critical job of organizing all the opinion reports furnished by the experts. There's the nephrologist's opinion on whether and when end-stage renal disease will begin and whether and when that will require dialysis or a kidney transplant. The physical and occupational therapists will furnish a report outlining future therapy needs. In the case of a child with HUS brought on by *E. coli* poisoning, the number of experts and reports goes on and on. Lawyers rely on the life-care planner to synthesize them all. Then an economist helps the lawyer figure out the projected costs for all the care.

Bill had one life-care planner handling the reports for Brianne and all of his other HUS cases. Anticipating one particular report that should have been completed sooner, Bill called the planner to find out what was holding up the show.

"Hey, it's Bill. When am I going to get that life-care plan from you?"

The life-care planner had a simple answer: as soon as he got paid for the previous life-care plan he had produced.

Bill didn't follow him.

"You guys haven't paid me for past work," the life-care planner put it directly.

"Look, I'm sure the bookkeeper just missed it," Bill told him. "I'll get this taken care of right away."

Bill walked down to the bookkeeper's office. "Hey, I need to get a check cut."

The bookkeeper burst into tears.

Bill took a step back, flashed a quizzical expression, and turned up the palms of his hands.

"I can't take this anymore," the bookkeeper cried, bolting from her desk.

"What the *hell?*" Bill said.

He went to Kargianis's office, figuring maybe he knew something since the bookkeeper had worked for him for some time. He asked if Kargianis knew what was wrong with her.

"What do you mean?" Kargianis asked.

Bill told him what had just happened.

Kargianis downplayed the outburst, suggesting the bookkeeper was probably just having a bad day.

A bad day? There had to be more to it than that. Bill went to see Osborn; maybe he knew something. But Osborn was out.

Luckily, Watkins was in. Bill ducked into Watkins's office and shut the door.

"Mike, what's going on?"

Watkins hesitated.

Bill raised his eyebrows, waiting for a response.

Watkins told Bill to have a seat. "We're over a $1 million under water," he said softly.

"What? What'd you say?"

"We're over a $1 million under water," Watkins repeated slowly.

Bill sprung to his feet. "Holy shit!"

Watkins grimaced and nodded his head up and down.

Bill didn't understand how that was possible. Kargianis was one of the more successful trial lawyers in Seattle. He and Osborn had come from one of the bigger plaintiffs' firms in the city. They were driving luxury cars, dressing to the nines, and occupying some of the most prized office space in Seattle. How in the *hell* could the firm be unable to afford a modest payment to a life-care planner?

Watkins knew how. But for Bill to understand he had to go back a few steps to the breakup of the big firm that Kargianis and Osborn had come from.

The business structure of most law firms is a partnership. When a partnership breaks up, it's not unusual for it to have debt, which becomes the responsibility of the individual partners.

"George paid a shitload of money in the outgoing of his old firm," Watkins explained. "George was in debt."

Naturally, that debt followed Kargianis when he and Osborn continued to work together in a much smaller firm, which got further behind in payments to expert witnesses, independent contractors, and vendors that supplied office computers, copy machines, and stationery. Even the office staff sometimes wondered whether their paychecks were going to bounce.

"And they rented space to me," Watkins explained, "because I was leaving the insurance-defense firm I'd been with for a long time. So I'm physically in their office. Then Sim comes to me at some point and says that he's walking down the street and he sees Bill, and Bill was a little blue about how Keller Rohrback is digging in their heels. He wants to be a partner, and he has the biggest case in the state of Washington. And Sim, who is very astute on the business side of the practice of law, realized, 'How could you go wrong if you partner up with the guy whose got the biggest case in the state of Washington?'"

Bill suddenly felt ill. He had promised to give these guys 60 percent of whatever fees he received on the *Kiner* case and any other *Jack in the Box* cases. He was starting to feel pretty stupid.

But there was more.

When Watkins and Marler joined forces with Kargianis and Osborn, the new firm used all the same vendors and experts and office staff that Kargianis and Osborn had been using. Some of them had not been paid for contracts and work performed before Bill came on board. Now those debts were Bill's problem, too.

"Shit, Mike, did you know this when I was negotiating with you guys to join your firm?"

"I knew we had problems. But I didn't understand the depth of this."

Bill covered his face with his hands and breathed in deeply. He exhaled, sliding his hands down his cheeks to his chin. He'd finally become a partner and all of a sudden he felt as if he'd met the Wizard of Oz. Badly in need of a stiff drink, he staggered out of Watkins's office.

That night Bill panicked.

"What the hell have I gotten myself into?" he said to Julie. "I don't know what to do."

Julie wasn't used to that. Bill always knew what to do in a crisis. It worried her to see him so worried.

Bill feared that the firm's financial woes would prevent him from delivering on his promises to the Kiners and the other clients from the Jack in the Box litigation that had severed their ties to Keller Rohrback. He wasn't about to end up on the hook for financial problems that had been present before he arrived. "This is bullshit," Bill said impulsively. "I'm leaving!"

It was simple—his new partners had dug themselves into a financial hole. They could dig themselves out.

But leaving his new firm two months after leaving his old firm wasn't that simple. What about the clients? The Kiners and the others had just withdrawn from Keller Rohrback and followed Bill to his new firm. If he informed them he was changing horses again, they'd surely start to question his stability. Not a good idea. *You are only as good as the clients that you have.* A seasoned personal-injury lawyer once said that to Bill. Now he appreciated what that meant.

There was another problem—even if he did leave, where would he go? It wasn't as if he had the resources to start up his own private practice.

It felt as if the walls were closing in on him. He had no choice but stay. "Damn it!"

_____

No one doubted that the honeymoon was over at Kargianis, Osborn, Watkins & Marler. The four lawyers filed into the conference room at their offices for some tough talk. A review of their individual caseloads revealed that all of them had plenty of clients. It was time to do everything possible to close cases and collect payments. In the meantime, office expenses had to be cut drastically. But they were locked into their expensive office lease. Cutting office staff wasn't an option either. That left partner compensation. All four of them agreed they'd go without a paycheck until the firm was in the black.

Bill's partners were better positioned to withstand an income suspension than he was. They were much more established and had more assets to leverage for personal loans: large homes, expensive cars, investments, and the like. Bill had none of that. And he and Julie had a baby and a monthly mortgage payment they were already struggling to make. Suddenly Bill was looking at a year or more before he'd draw a paycheck from the firm. It could easily take that long to settle the *Jack in the Box* cases.

Desperate, Bill went to see an old friend, Dick Krutch. He was a very successful aviation lawyer. Back when Bill had been going through his divorce, he had rented an apartment from Krutch. They had become close. Krutch was considerably older than Bill and took on the role of mentor. After law school Bill had trouble finding a job. Desperate, he approached Krutch, who hired him to work on a big lawsuit he had against Boeing. Krutch represented a woman who lost her husband and son when Japan Airlines Flight 123 crashed near Mount Osutaka after suffering mechanical failure. Only four of the 509 passengers survived. It was the worst air disaster in history. Krutch prevailed, and Bill learned invaluable lessons about how to prepare a case for trial.

Now he went to Krutch with a simple plea: "I need a loan."

Krutch had a longstanding relationship with a banker. With Krutch's backing, the banker agreed to provide Bill and Julie a sixty-thousand-dollar personal line of credit and money for the firm if needed. It would serve as a substitute for Bill's lost annual salary.

Once that was in place, Bill told Julie that this Christmas would be different, as in, he'd be working. Trials were approaching. Bills had to be paid. Experts had to be retained. Clients needed attention. "There's a lot of shit I have to worry about," he said. "I just have to work myself out of this mess."

Julie got it. When she had married Bill she'd been under no illusions about his work habits. She was fine with that. He was happier when he was buried in work.

Bill told her that in addition to handling the entire Jack in the Box litigation on his own, he also planned to take over the management of his law firm. That was something he knew nothing about. To get himself up to speed, he adopted a new daily schedule:

- Arise at 4:30 a.m.
- Catch the 5:25 a.m. ferry from Bainbridge Island to Seattle.
- Arrive at the office at 6:15 a.m.
- Leave the office at 8:15 p.m.
- Catch the 8:40 p.m. ferry back to the island.
- Arrive home just before 9:30 p.m.

Saturdays and Sundays were no exception.
Julie's response to all this was simple: whatever it takes.

37

THE NEW NORMAL

January 31, 1994

LAWYERS DON'T NORMALLY VISIT THE HOMES OF THEIR CLIENTS. BUT nothing about the *Kiner* case was normal. That suited Bill just fine. He never liked doing things the way everyone else did. So when Suzanne invited him to Brianne's eleventh birthday party, Bill didn't hesitate.

Without notifying the family, he hired a clown and dispatched him to the Kiner home. When Bill arrived, he was pleased to find the clown entertaining Brianne and all of her former classmates from her old elementary school. Although she had been home from the hospital for seven months, Brianne was still not capable of returning to school. Doctors advised that she'd probably never return to grammar school. There were just too many medical impediments. An in-home tutor had been assigned instead. Fortunately, Brianne's schoolmates remained her friends.

Bill ducked inside and faded into the background. Brianne looked so much better than the first time he had met her, in the ICU. Just the fact that she was celebrating a birthday was a remarkable milestone. In many respects, the party was like any other eleven-year-old's birthday party. There were games, gifts, and cake and ice cream. But Bill couldn't help noticing the differences—the presence of nurses and a lawyer looking on, symptoms of the new normal in Brianne's life.

Keller Rohrback and Chris Pence were bearing down. Bill had heard from more than one lawyer that his old firm had been asking around, trying to find out if Bill had approached other firms besides Kargianis & Osborn and dangled the *Kiner* case in exchange for a partnership. Bill hadn't. But just the fact that Keller Rohrback was fishing for this kind of information was proof that they were digging in for a fight. Bill knew his new firm was in no condition to sustain a battle with his old one.

He and Watkins had been working with an accountant and a paralegal to take a closer look at the firm's finances. What they found alarmed them. The firm wasn't just in debt; the record keeping was in shambles. Unpaid invoices were everywhere. Receipts weren't filed. Debits and assets hadn't been properly tracked. A forensic accountant would have easily declared the books a disaster.

Worse, client files were in disarray. There was so much to do that Bill knew he needed a quick way out of the Keller Rohrback dispute. He figured the best way was to see if Keller Rohrback would agree to mediation. Watkins thought that made a lot of sense. Bill knew whom to call.

Judicial Arbitration & Mediation Services (JAMS) was started in Seattle by a group of judges who retired from the bench and set up a for-fee service to resolve disputes out of court. Judge Gerald Shellan was one of the first judges to join JAMS. A Columbia Law School graduate, Shellan started practicing law in 1950 and remained in private practice until he joined the bench in 1977. He became the presiding judge in King County Superior Court in 1982. Complex business litigation and marriage dissolution were among his specialty areas. But that wasn't why Bill recommended using Shellan to mediate his dispute with Keller Rohrback. He wanted Shellan because he'd clerked for him back when he was in law school, and he was convinced that his reputation for fairness and reasonableness was unsurpassed.

Even Keller Rohrback and Pence couldn't argue with the selection of Shellan. But they were prepared to argue about everything else, especially money. Surely a guy duplicitous and disloyal enough to steal the *Kiner* case would come into the negotiations determined to hold on to as much of the fee from that case as possible. "He made a very calculated decision based on his financial interests," Pence explained.

In advance of the mediation, Bill received a copy of the mediation letter that Keller Rohrback and Pence had submitted to Judge Shellan. It outlined the complaint against Bill, accusing him of violating numerous provisions from the code of conduct set for lawyers by the Washington State Bar Association. The gist of it was that Bill stole clients. The unmistakable threat behind the complaint was that if Bill didn't pay up, he'd be sued.

Bill showed the document to his new law partners. They weren't eager to see Bill settle, not if settling meant agreeing to give his old firm a cut of the legal fees that would eventually be generated by the *Kiner* case and the other HUS cases that had followed Bill to his new law firm. Kargianis, Osborn, and Watkins were poised to collect 60 percent of those fees. Their cut would be diminished if some of those fees went to Keller Rohrback and Chris Pence. So their reaction to the letter was simple: "Tell them to go to hell."

Despite his partners' attitude, Bill had no intention of fighting. He went to see Brad Keller for advice. After reading Keller Rohrback's mediation letter, Keller assured Bill that most of it—especially the stuff claiming Bill had violated Washington's code of conduct for lawyers—was just lawyers blowing smoke. On the other hand, Keller said, Bill's old law firm was undoubtedly entitled to a portion of the fees from the cases that had originated in their offices. *Quantum meruit* is a legal doctrine that implies a promise to pay a reasonable amount for the labor and materials furnished. Clearly, Keller Rohrback had invested some resources and manpower in the very early stages of these cases. For that, the firm deserved compensation.

"The question," Keller explained, "is how do you go about determining what is fair and appropriate?"

Bill pointed out that nobody else at Keller Rohrback had had any real contact with the Kiner family or the other clients. This was generally true of the handful of other Jack in the Box clients that had followed Bill to his new firm. Since none of these clients were included in the class-action suit, Bill had done virtually all of the work on their cases. So for the firm to seek a big cut of the fees generated from these cases didn't seem fair.

Keller agreed.

There was another thing to think about. Bill had left Keller Rohrback right after Suzanne Kiner had signed the retainer agreement. The fact was that very little work had been done on the *Kiner* case at Keller Rohrback. The overwhelming majority of work on that case was still in front of Bill, not behind him. So his old law firm really shouldn't have been entitled to very much.

Keller generally agreed with that, too.

Bill assured him he wasn't in the mood to argue anyway. "At this point, I have enough distractions," he said, explaining that his top priority was making the dispute with Keller Rohrback and Chris Pence vanish. "I'm just going to give up more than I think I should give up."

Keller saw some wisdom in this approach, assuring him that he was smart to pay more money to get rid of a problem.

"I'm willing to do that to avoid a side show," Bill told Keller.

38

THE RECKONING

May 11, 1994

IT WAS AFTER 10:00 P.M. WHEN BILL SLID INTO BED. LYING ON HIS BACK, he stared up into the darkness, his heart pounding hard and rapidly. His chest felt constricted. *What the hell have I gotten myself into?*

He and Julie were falling behind on bills. Julie had gone back to work part-time and was pulling in just enough to pay for groceries. Bill's mother was helping out with child care. All of these problems had started when Bill left Keller Rohrback, which was now primed to sue him.

I can't believe I've gotten my wife and kid in this spot. He felt sweaty and his breathing was labored.

Suddenly Julie rolled over and saddled up close to him. She knew what he was thinking. "Don't worry about it," she said. "We'll figure this out."

The Next Day
JAMS Offices
Seattle, Washington

Judge Shellan had no idea what he was in for, but it didn't take him long to find out. A pipe-smoking, coffee-drinking man with silver hair and an expression of father-knows-best, Shellan welcomed both parties to the JAMS offices. Bill was accompanied by Mike Watkins. Keller Rohrback had sent a small contingency of lawyers led by Kirk Portman, a senior partner whom Bill knew fairly well. Pence was with them. Sarko had desperately wanted to attend, but he'd left town a month earlier to begin the *Exxon Valdez* trial in Alaska.

With the parties all together, Shellan reminded everyone why they were there, and he mapped out the procedure that he planned to follow. Then he ushered the parties into separate rooms and met privately with each side. The hard part was figuring out how much the *Kiner* case was worth. Up to that point, the largest personal-injury award in Washington State history had been $10 million. Neither side expected the *Kiner* case to reach eight figures. But anywhere between $1 million and $9 million was possible. The problem was that the bigger the pot of money, the more a tort lawyer wants.

Eventually, Pence and Portman proposed a fee arrangement that would work on a sliding scale. So, for example, if the Kiner case settled for an amount between $1 million and $5 million, they'd be entitled to a certain percentage. They'd be entitled to a lesser percentage if *Kiner* settled for somewhere between $5 million and $7.5 million. And anything over $7.5 million would yield an even lower percentage.

Bill agreed to this approach and the rest of the day was spent trying to refine the dollar amounts and the percentages. The two sides appeared on the verge of agreement when Shellan brought in the final written proposal from Pence and Portman. It wasn't until Bill and Watkins saw the numbers on paper that they realized the two sides were actually miles apart.

All along, Bill and Watkins had assumed the percentage owed would decrease as the gross settlement fee rose. So if *Kiner* settled for $5 million, the fee might be split fifty-fifty with Keller Rohrback. If Kiner settled for $7.5 million, Keller Rohrback might receive only 40 percent of the fee, and so forth. But Pence and Portman wanted 50 percent of the first $5 million and 40 percent of the next $2.5 million.

As soon as Shellan reported the discrepancy to Pence and Portman, the negotiations immediately went south. "I thought Bill lacked a moral center, a moral compass," Pence recalled. "Remember, at this point money was an issue. I don't think I said: 'That bastard just stole the biggest case.' I don't remember that. But I'm not saying I'm unaffected by my financial interests. I am affected by my financial interests."

When Shellan returned to Bill's room and told him the news, Bill fell silent.

Fed up, Watkins rose to his feet and started packing his briefcase. "Big deal if they sue us," he announced. "We're professional litigators."

Figuring it was over, Shellan headed for the door.

"Wait," Bill said softly, freezing Shellan. "Hold on a minute."

Shellan looked at him. Bill's cheeks were red and his eyes were welling up. It was clear he needed a moment. Shellan said he'd be waiting outside.

Bill sat like a boulder, still and silent. Some lawyers need a dispute the same way people need a drink in their hand at a party. Without one they seem purposeless. Not Bill. To him conflict was anathema. It didn't accomplish anything. That was why he'd come in prepared to pay his former colleagues whatever it took to satisfy them, even if it meant swallowing hard and giving Keller Rohrback more than he felt they deserved. Still, that was better than the alternative—protracted litigation.

The one thing he wasn't prepared for, however, was being forced to swallow his pride. From Bill's perspective, Pence wouldn't even be working with Keller Rohrback on the *Jack in the Box* case if Bill hadn't come up with idea of a merger while helping Pence move one weekend. For that matter, Keller Rohrback wouldn't have a class-action suit with

---

Through mediation, Bill Marler settled the dispute with his old firm while simultaneously litigating against Jack in the Box and trying to keep his new firm from going under.

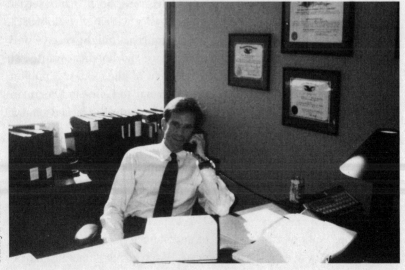

two hundred clients if Bill hadn't brought in the first case and gotten the ball rolling and done the media groundwork to reign in so many others. Plus, it was Bill's relationship with Piper that had convinced Piper to make Keller Rohrback the preferred choice to get control of the class once it was certified by the court.

Bill took a deep breath and gathered himself.

"I just don't give a shit about the money," Bill told Watkins.

Watkins was starting to understand. But he still didn't want to give in. To him this was about principle—if this thing went to court, Watkins insisted, Keller Rohrback would get much less than Bill was offering it. So let the bastards sue.

"Mike, it just ain't worth it to fight about this."

Watkins dropped his chin and let out a sigh. He asked Bill what he wanted to do.

"If it means I have to give up more to Keller Rohrback than I think they're entitled to, then I'm willing to do that. We've got to get this behind us."

Watkins capitulated. "We need to settle this," he agreed.

Bill motioned for Shellan to come back in. Then he told him what he was prepared to offer Keller Rohrback on the *Kiner* case:

- Fifty percent of the fee on the first $8 million.

- One-third of the fee from $8 million to $10 million.

- Twenty-five percent of any fee in excess of $10 million.

Shellan raised his eyebrows.

Bill wasn't through. He also offered to pay his former law firm one-third of the fees he generated on every other *E. coli* case he settled.

As soon as Shellan walked next door and shared the offer with the other side, all the shouting stopped. The game was over.

"I remember being surprised at how favorable the settlement was to us," Pence reflected later. "I was surprised. That has put him in good standing. He built a ton of goodwill by being so fair with money."

Both parties signed the agreement. Keller Rohrback got what it was after—money. And Bill was free to advocate for the Kiner family the way he saw fit.

39

THE SUGGESTION BOX

DENIS STEARNS HAD COMPLETED HIS AUDIT OF JACK IN THE BOX'S internal files, and he didn't like what he had found. Piper wanted a complete rundown. Stearns began with the issue of internal cooking temperatures for beef.

Back when Washington State had upped the mandatory cooking temperatures to 155 degrees as a way to kill *E. coli* in meat, it hadn't limited the safety changes to beef. The state had also increased the minimum cooking temperature for chicken, Stearns said.

Piper found this interesting. But he wasn't sure why this was relevant.

"Back before the outbreak," Stearns explained, "Jack in the Box started making changes to its operations manuals to elevate the internal cooking temperature for chicken." This suggested that the company had known a lot more about the rule change than it had let on. Stearns said he was convinced that people in the company had known.

Piper didn't get it. If they had known and they had gone through the trouble of increasing their cooking temperatures in chicken to be in compliance with Washington State law, why had they not done the same thing for beef?

Stearns had a theory. Back before the outbreak, Ken Dunkley had called for a massive survey of all state health department regulations in an effort to see which ones were at odds with the company's operations manual for restaurant managers. A draft of the results had reached

Dunkley's desk before the outbreak. "Whether he was consciously aware of the cooking-temperature change and whether its significance occurred to him, no one will ever know," Stearns said. "We know that the cooking-temperature change regarding chicken had been acted on, but my guess is that this was triggered independent of Dunkley's regulation-review process."

Stearns felt confident in this conclusion after spending so much time studying the fast-food chain's internal corporate structure. The company bought and sold so much chicken and beef that chicken and beef products were handled by different people within the company. And each one had responsibility for its own sections of the operating manual. It was very understandable that one group of employees in the corporate office could have acted on the notice from Washington State to raise meat-cooking temperatures while the other one wouldn't have. It's the kind of thing that could easily happen when the business of feeding people was set up like a giant chain of retail stores.

"The folks in charge of chicken viewed it as a more dangerous product," Stearns explained. "Remember, prior to the outbreak, hamburger was just not considered that dangerous. So I don't think Dunkley knowingly failed to pass on information that he understood to be of significance. He was just being methodical and slow, without any sense of urgency because it was 'only' fast food after all. What could go wrong?"

Piper thought Stearns's explanation made a lot of sense. But he was sure that this scenario wouldn't play well in front of a Seattle jury. Poisoned consumers would have no sympathy for the notion that Jack in the Box was such a big corporation that one hand didn't know what the other one was doing. Marler was going to have a field day with this information. After all, Jack in the Box had been stating all along that it hadn't known about Washington's new law. Well, it had known enough to raise the cooking temperature for chicken. At best, the company looked negligent by not having done the same for beef. Marler, Piper figured, would insist this had been by design in order to insure the preferred flavor in the hamburger patties.

There were other damaging discoveries, such as a file that the company maintained with feedback from local restaurant managers.

The feedback was transmitted through a standard form called In the Suggestion Box. One of these submissions particularly troubled Stearns. Back before the outbreak a number of Seattle-area restaurant managers had received customer complaints concerning hamburgers that were raw in the middle. One employee entered the following on her report to corporate headquarters:

> Describe Changes: I think regular patties should cook longer. They don't get done and we have customer complaints.
>
> Describe Benefit: If we change this we will be making our burgers done and edible.

After submitting this suggestion, the restaurant manager received a letter from corporate headquarters stating, "We would like to acknowledge the time and effort you have taken to contribute to the success of Jack in the Box by enclosing this pen/highlighter."

With evidence like this, Stearns felt it was going to be pretty hard for Jack in the Box to say that it hadn't known it had a problem with undercooking its beef patties.

Piper agreed. They had trouble on their hands.

Stearns raised a more immediate concern: Bill Marler. For months he had been filing broad document requests and for months Stearns had been limiting what got turned over to him. Now that Stearns had found all these potentially damning documents about increased cooking temperatures for chicken and complaints from customers and managers about undercooked hamburgers, he figured he had to turn them over proactively.

Piper didn't see a way around turning them over either.

But Stearns figured there was at least a way to make these documents hard for Marler to find—to send so much documentation that Marler would be overwhelmed. In other words, he would do what was known as a "document dump" on Marler. Send him thousands of documents and hope that he didn't find the few damaging ones.

Piper liked the idea and gave Stearns the go-ahead.

40

BINGO

FOR WEEKS BILL HAD BEEN HOLED UP IN A CONFERENCE ROOM, SURROUNDED by more than fifty banker boxes full of operations manuals, internal memos, and every other imaginable piece of paper generated by Jack in the Box. When the boxes had first arrived, Bill figured Piper and Stearns were betting that he'd never wade through so much material. Determined to prove them wrong, Bill spent months poring over each file. When he had assisted Dick Krutch in that air-disaster lawsuit against Boeing, Bill had learned a valuable lesson: personal-injury lawsuits were won and lost during discovery. The lawyer willing to invest the most time piecing together the paper trail was often the lawyer who prevailed. It boiled down to persistence. There were no shortcuts.

Relentless, Bill eventually found all the documents that implicated Jack in the Box, the ones that Stearns had brought to Piper's attention. Bill laughed when he found the memo that awarded a pen to the manager who said the restaurant's hamburgers would be edible if they were cooked longer. But he knew he had hit pay dirt when he discovered something more critical—an explanation for why only some of the Jack in the Box restaurants in the greater Seattle area were linked to sick kids during the outbreak. If all the beef at the central distribution center had been contaminated and all the restaurants had gotten their beef from the distribution center, then why had some of the restaurants escaped being linked to the outbreak? It was a question that had nagged him for a long time.

These internal documents from Jack in the Box helped Bill Marler build a case against the company.

In studying the operations manual, Bill saw that all the restaurants had been required to cook their beef patties for two minutes. But in looking at the restaurants that were linked to the outbreak, Bill realized that all of them were older establishments with older grills. The newer restaurants had newer equipment that tended to cook a couple of degrees higher. When it came to *E. coli*, a couple of degrees could be the difference between life and death.

It came down to this: on the newer grills, two minutes was sufficient to cook the center of the burger. But on the old grills, two minutes often left the burgers undercooked in the middle. In the end, none of this would have mattered had Jack in the Box simply adhered to the Washington State standard and cooked all of its hamburgers to an internal temperature of 155 degrees, although the new grills cooked hotter. Unfortunately, the two-minute cook times were geared to get the meat to an internal temperature of 140 degrees.

At an analytical level, Bill understood how a food-safety regulation could have fallen through the cracks at a big corporation. But on a human level, he knew that consumers deserved a higher standard of excellence when it came to product reliability. Eating, after all, wasn't a choice. And people entering a restaurant ought to have had the assurance that the food was being prepared in accordance with current safety standards.

Yet everyone from the beef processors to the regulators to the lawmakers had been too cavalier about *E. coli* O157:H7 for too long. Bill had become convinced that the best way to stop business-as-usual in the food industry was through external pressure. That meant extracting big damages awards out of Jack in the Box. The higher the numbers the more the industry would sit up and pay attention.

The *Kiner* case was by far Bill's best weapon. That was what had him worried. The *Kiner* case was only as strong as Suzanne. And Bill knew she was fragile. Most people would have cracked under all the stress she'd been shouldering. He just hoped she could hang on a little longer. He was starting to feel the finish line was almost in sight.

In hopes of speeding up the process, he wanted an updated, expanded video of Brianne and her condition. The idea was to show her trying to learn how to walk and talk again. This time he hired

Sim Osborn's wife, one of the most successful television journalists in Seattle.

Once the video was finished, Bill delivered copies to Piper. The message was clear: *If Jack in the Box doesn't do right by Brianne and this case ends up going to trial, these images are what you can expect a jury to see.*

41

TURNING POINT

July 1994

ABC News had spent a long time investigating the *E. coli* outbreak in Seattle. It had also been looking into broader questions about meat safety and the federal regulations that govern it. All the research was coming together for a hard-hitting segment on *Turning Point*. The network hired Emmy Award–winning documentary filmmaker Michael Mierendorf to produce and direct the segment. Meredith Vieira, a tough journalist who had recently been at *60 Minutes*, was assigned as the correspondent. ABC had spent a great deal of time with Dave Theno, visiting restaurants and meat plants. But what the show was really after was a sit-down interview with Nugent.

The prospect of facing off with Vieira made Nugent very wary. He discussed it with Theno, who agreed that it was a bad idea. "She's very, very tough," Theno said. "She can chew you up and spit you out."

A public relations firm working for Jack in the Box agreed. There just didn't appear to be anything good coming out of *Turning Point*'s story. The expectation was that over 10 million viewers might tune in to an episode that was sure to cast a less than flattering light on Jack in the Box and ground beef. The fast-food chain was already struggling to stay afloat. This was the sort of thing that could sink the company.

But Jack in the Box also realized that *Turning Point* was going to do the story with or without Nugent's participation. The PR team reasoned that it probably made more sense to participate and at least try to tell the restaurant's side. The good news was that more than a year and a half had passed since the outbreak, and during that time the company had implemented a food-safety system that was a model for the entire industry. Nugent finally agreed to go along after a member of the company's corporate communications team came up with a clever idea: to send along an in-house videographer to film ABC filming Nugent. The hope was to keep ABC honest. With an outside camera in the room, *Turning Point* would be less likely to take things out of context, and if it did, the restaurant chain would have the footage to make its case.

The night before the interview was to take place in Seattle, Nugent flew up with Theno. They spent the night in a Seattle hotel and had agreed to meet in the hotel's restaurant for breakfast. When Theno entered the restaurant the following morning, he found Nugent had already taken a table. Nugent told Theno that he had bumped into Meredith Vieira a few minutes earlier.

"What was *that* like?" Theno asked.

"She couldn't have been sweeter," Nugent said, admitting he had been pretty apprehensive when he approached her. He told Theno that Vieira had smiled and shaken his hand and that they had talked very briefly about their children. It had been a brief encounter, but Nugent was at ease. One more thing . . . Vieira was even prettier in person than on television.

Theno wasn't surprised that Vieira looked even better up close. But he had his doubts about her sweetness. "Bob, I have to tell you, these people can be absolutely brutal," Theno warned. "They can smile at you and eviscerate you at the same time."

After that, Nugent didn't feel much like eating.

The location of the interview was a brand-new Jack in the Box restaurant outside Seattle. Michael Mierendorf and his crew got there hours beforehand to set the stage. The restaurant was closed to customers. Tables and chairs were cleared out of the dining area, replaced by cords, cables, microphones, spotlights, and cameras. By the time Nugent and Theno arrived, the restaurant looked like a television studio. Although Nugent's company owned the property, he felt as if he had entered enemy territory. The tension in the room was palpable as an entourage of Jack in the Box staff crowded around the outside of the set. More than a dozen ABC crew members were in place, some of them standing around with their arms folded. That was when Jack in the Box's videographer began to set up his camera. Mierendorf had had no idea this was coming, and he wasn't happy.

"He just showed up," Mierendorf explained. "It was a new one on me. I didn't like it."

The awkward stand-off made the atmosphere even more nerve-racking. Before long, Mierendorf threw up his hands. "There was nothing we could do about it," he explained. "What could we do, pack our bags and go home?"

Vieira, wearing a stylish black jacket, took a seat at one of the restaurant tables. Nugent sat opposite her with a Jack in the Box soft drink cup in his hand. He looked relaxed. But he wasn't. The bright lights made him uncomfortable. It was all he could do not to squint. Vieira's first couple of questions weren't particularly difficult. But it

Bob Nugent being interviewed by Meredith Vieira for
ABC's Turning Point.

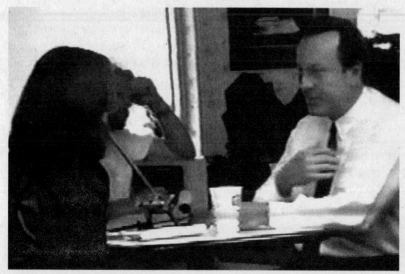

Courtesy of Bill Marler

didn't take long for her direct style to start getting under Nugent's skin. He felt like he was being interrogated.

"Do you believe now in retrospect that Jack in the Box chose not to pay attention to certain things, like the law?" she asked.

"No, I don't believe that at all," Nugent said. "We would never choose not to pay attention to the law. Why would a company choose not to pay attention to the law?"

"I don't know," Vieira said.

"We are not only a proud company and a quality . . . a company that's concerned with quality, but we're a moral company, too," Nugent said.

Vieira challenged that. She knew that after the outbreak had been announced in Seattle, kids had started getting sick with *E. coli* in Nevada. And state health officials there had had no idea that some of Jack in the Box's tainted meat had made it into their state. But Jack in the Box had known it.

"Did you notify health departments—" Vieira began.

"Well," Nugent interrupted.

"—as you were pulling that from the system?" she continued.

"You know, I don't have good recall on that."

Vieira continued to press Nugent about the company's failure to notify health officials in Nevada about bad meat there.

"The last thing we wanted to do was to set a panic, an alarm, that there was a problem when in fact there wasn't," Nugent said. "We had no idea whether or not the product had been sold."

"But how is that creating a problem, to tell health officials?" Vieira asked. "I think that would be preventing the problem. I would think that would be information you would want to share."

Nugent was befuddled. "Well, there . . . you . . . there's . . . that's a good point. And I . . . and perhaps we should have done that."

Looking on, Theno dropped his head. "Oh shit," he murmured under his breath. Nugent had been given some perfunctory media training, but nothing to prepare him for this.

Vieira kept coming. Irritated, Nugent started rubbing his finger across the rim of his water glass. An ABC crewmember said they were picking up some interference in Nugent's microphone and asked if he could refrain from rubbing the glass. Nugent stood up and asked to be excused. The cameras cut off as Nugent walked over to the kitchen, where Theno and Nugent's publicist had congregated.

"We're getting the *hell* outta here," Nugent said.

"Bob, you're doing great," the publicist reassured him.

Nugent didn't want to hear it. He felt completely blindsided and wished he had trusted his initial instincts to avoid this interview altogether. "I am *not* going through with this," Nugent said.

"You *have* to go through with it," the publicist insisted, saying you just didn't walk away from a network television interview with Meredith Vieira. "We'll look like fools if you don't go back."

Theno had disagreed with the initial decision to have Nugent do the interview. But now that they were on the set, he agreed with the publicist. It was too late to turn back.

Nugent fumed. "This is going to come back to bite us in the ass," he said.

Then he reached for the phone and called back to corporate headquarters in San Diego. Before going any further with Vieira he wanted to talk to the legal department.

"We needed to let them know how it was going and see if there was any damage control that needed to be done," Theno explained.

As Mierendorf watched Nugent talking on the telephone, he couldn't help wondering what was up. *Was Nugent going to walk out?*

One thing was clear: Jack in the Box had not expected Vieira to be so well prepared. "I didn't think Meredith badgered him," Mierendorf explained. "She *pushed* him. But she didn't badger him. We knew more than he thought we'd know."

Finally, Nugent returned. When he sat down, Vieira asked him if he wanted to redo some of the earlier sequences. The gesture seemed to take the edge off. But by the time the interview finally wrapped up, everyone involved felt drained.

"It was becoming increasingly clear to me as we produced this thing exactly what was at stake for everybody involved," Mierendorf explained. "This is the sort of thing that is potentially ruinous for companies. So we better be right and we better be fair."

Nugent left the restaurant in disgust. He couldn't help directing some of his anger at Vieira. He compared her to Jekyll and Hyde. But most of his indignation was directed at himself. He was exceptional at a lot of things. But prime time television interviews weren't among them. He felt like he'd let his company down by not doing a better job defending its record.

On the car ride back to the hotel, Theno tried to reassure him. Not even an experienced talking head, he insisted, could have held up well under that kind of questioning. He suggested the two of them go to a bar. "I'm buying," Theno said.

"Well then I'm drinking," Nugent said.

ABC aired Meredith Vieira's interview with Nugent on *Turning Point* on October 12, 1994. The segment was titled: "Deadly Meat: When a Hamburger Can Kill." The show opened with Vieira asking the viewers a question: "Could eating a hamburger kill your child?"

Bill Marler was watching from home with a remote control in his hand and a VHS tape running in his VCR. He recorded the whole program, thinking it might give him some fodder for his upcoming deposition of Nugent. In that respect, the program didn't disappoint. But Bill had done enough television interviews to know that most of what you say never makes it on the air. A one-hour interview can result in a thirty-second sound bite. He couldn't help wondering what else Nugent had said that had ended up on the cutting room floor.

The next day he called ABC News in New York and requested the unedited video footage of the entire interview Vieira did with Nugent. When Mierendorf learned of Bill's request, he couldn't help thinking that this lawyer was pretty ingenious. It also occurred to him that what goes around comes around.

A lawyer in ABC's legal department promptly rejected Bill's request. Bill countered by threatening to subpoena the footage. ABC's attorney scoffed, informing Bill that the material was protected by the

First Amendment. That issue had been decided by the U.S. Supreme Court. The lawyer invited Bill to look it up.

The get-tough approach wasn't working. Bill tried a different tack—friendly conversation. A few minutes later they were still talking. Eventually the ABC lawyer softened. "You know," the lawyer said, "Jack in the Box was filming us filming Nugent."

Bill paused. "They did *what*? They filmed it *themselves*?"

As soon as he hung up the phone, Bill roared with laughter and ran down the hallway to tell anyone he could find, "You'll never believe this one. . . ."

Then he placed a call to Denis Stearns.

"*You* guys filmed that?" Bill said, making no effort to hide his pleasure.

"*We* didn't!" Stearns said defensively. "The Foodmaker people did."

"Well, I want it. I want all of it."

Stearns wanted to tell Marler to go to hell. But he couldn't. Marler was entitled to a copy. Stearns just couldn't believe that Marler had found out about it. No other trial lawyer with cases against Jack in the Box had thought to call ABC, much less get the news organization to cough up the information.

Stearns was sure of one thing. Whoever had had the bright idea to tape Nugent's interview should be fired. ABC had actually been kind to Jack in the Box by not airing some of the exchanges between Vieira and Nugent that made the executive look like he was either lying or utterly incompetent. Marler, Stearns feared, would pounce once he got his hands on this stuff.

42

THE DEPOSITION

Wednesday, November 16, 1994
San Diego

WEARING BRAND NEW SHOES AND A PRESSED SUIT, BILL FILED INTO A large conference room at the downtown law offices of Gibson, Dunn & Crutcher. Facing a video camera, Bob Nugent was seated beside Denis Stearns and a court reporter. Seven other lawyers were on hand to observe Nugent's deposition, including two attorneys representing Vons and one representing a consortium of meat-packing companies.

Bill politely shook their hands. But he had only one thing on his mind. In all of Nugent's public statements, he had remained adamantly consistent about two things: First, that prior to the outbreak he'd never heard of *E. coli*, and second, that he'd had no idea that Washington State had raised the internal cooking temperatures on beef to 155 degrees. This was the story that he'd told Congress, Meredith Vieira, and anyone else who would listen. He had even gone a step further, insisting that prior to the outbreak *no one in his company* had known about *E. coli* or the new law in Washington.

Bill's mission was straightforward—to establish that Nugent *should* have known both those things. With the reporter and the videographer ready, Bill and Nugent faced each other.

"Mr. Nugent, my name is Bill Marler. I represent three children who became injured as a result of ingesting *E. coli* O157:H7–tainted hamburger meat purchased at your restaurants in the Seattle area. I'm here today to ask questions of you on their behalf."

Steely-eyed, Nugent showed no expression.

UNITED STATES DISTRICT COURT

WESTERN DISTRICT OF WASHINGTON

AT SEATTLE

In re FOODMAKER/) NO. C93-161Z and
JACK-IN-THE-BOX LITIGATION) related cases
)

DEPOSITION OF ROBERT J. NUGENT

Wednesday, November 16, 1994
San Diego, California

****** ******

BYERS & ANDERSON, INC.

COURT REPORTING AND RECORDS COLLECTION

2208 North 30th Street   First Interstate Center
Suite 202   999 Third Avenue
Tacoma, Washington 98403   Suite 3210
(206) 627-6401   Seattle, Washington 98104
Fax: (206) 383-4884   (206) 340-1316

1

y objection interposed by a

all defendants unless

REPORTER: Sir, I'll go

ou raise your right hand.

ng been first duly sworn by

Notary, deposed and

tified as follows:

ION

arler and I met you just

ition. I represent three

s a result of ingesting

rger meat purchased at your

ea in Washington.

uestions of you on their

a question that you do not

is compound or if it's a

making myself clear, I'd

"Bill, you know, slow down

23   and stop or, you know, let's do something different."

24   And feel free to do that at any time, because I want

25   your testimony to be clear and understandable, and I

Robert J. Nugent by Mr. Marler - 11/16/94   8

A copy of the transcript of Bill Marler's deposition of Bob Nugent.

Bill breezed through the particulars about the spelling of Nugent's name, his home address, his professional background, and his title with the company. He was eager to get to the chain of command and who had known what when.

"Okay," Bill said. "Mo Iqbal. What is his role or what was his role prior to the outbreak, and is that role the same as it is today?"

"Mo was the head of marketing for Jack in the Box."

"And what does he do today?"

"He's not with our company."

Stearns held his breath. It was true that Iqbal no longer worked for Jack in the Box. But he still had close ties to Foodmaker, which had a 39-percent stake in Family Restaurants, Inc., where Iqbal held the title of president. The deposition would go sideways really fast if Marler started pushing down that path.

But Bill was focused on nailing down who in the chain of command had known about the 155-degree rule. He asked about Dunkley.

"Mr. Dunkley reported to Mo Iqbal," Nugent said.

"Okay. And then Mr. Iqbal would report to you?"

"That's correct."

Under questioning, Nugent confirmed that he had met regularly with Iqbal to discuss quality assurance of food products.

Bill directed Nugent to watch a clip from his interview with Meredith Vieira. It was an exchange that wasn't seen by the television audience.

Nugent: We knew about O157:H7. What we didn't know was how very virulent, how very powerful this particular bacteria was. I think that was common knowledge in the industry.

Vieira: What was common knowledge?

Nugent: That nobody had an understanding of just how powerful this particular bacteria was.

Bill stopped the tape. "The question I have for you, Mr. Nugent, is when did you personally know of the virulent strain of *E. coli* bacteria O157:H7?"

"During the week of January the 18th, 1993."

"So is it your testimony today that prior to that time you did not have any knowledge of the *E. coli* O157:H7 bacteria?

"Yes, that's correct."

"As you sit here today, do you know whether or not anyone in the Foodmaker organization knew of the *E. coli* O157:H7 bacterium prior to January 18, 1993?"

"No one knew."

"In reviewing the tape that we just saw, it was my understanding that what you were saying was that you knew of the bacteria prior to the date of January 18th, 1993."

Nugent asked Bill to rewind the tape far enough back to see the question that solicited his answer. Bill did that.

Vieira: Two questions come to mind: Where was Jack in the Box during all those hearings when the Department of Health said that it was notified, "Please come, please participate; this law affects you as a restaurant owner (of) over a thousand restaurants?" And where were your quality-assurance people who should keep up with the law? I mean, yeah, granted the Department of Health should send out notification, but where are all these quality-assurance people who should be on top of things?"

Nugent: Well, we knew about O157:H7. . . ."

Bill stopped the tape and looked at Nugent. "Mr. Nugent, is it still your testimony that when you were speaking to this reporter that you were indicating to her that your knowledge about *E. coli* O157:H7 did not predate January 18, 1993?"

Nugent shook his head. "I see the tape. I . . . I am frankly baffled. I can tell you, sitting here today, that prior to January 1993, it is my understanding that our people did not . . . were not aware of O157:H7 as being a bacteria that would . . . could be in our products and do the kinds of things that it did."

This was exactly the kind of thing that Stearns was afraid of: Marler making Nugent out to be a *baffled* chief executive. That wouldn't play well in front of a jury, not when little children were dead.

"Is it your testimony also that your people did not know of the *E. coli* O157:H7 bacteria?" Bill asked.

Stearns objected. "The question is calling for speculation."

After being advised by Stearns, Nugent said that within days of the outbreak he personally asked Ken Dunkley if he'd ever heard of O157:H7 and his response was no.

Bill pounced. "Mr. Nugent, do you receive the *Los Angeles Times?*"

"Pardon me?" Nugent said, caught off guard by the question.

"Do you receive the *Los Angeles Times?*"

"No."

"Does Jack in the Box receive the *Los Angeles Times*, San Diego edition?"

"I don't know, but I'm sure there are individuals within the company that do."

Bill handed him an exhibit marked F-29. "It is a *Los Angeles Times* newspaper dated July 11, 1990."

Nugent glanced at it.

"I ask you to look at the upper left-hand corner."

The headline read: "Battling an Elusive Bacterium."

Nugent admitted that this story had not come to his attention until his lawyers showed it to him in preparation for his deposition.

"Okay," Bill said. "Handing you what's been marked as F-52. I'll ask you if you have seen this document."

Nugent gave it a cursory look. "I have not."

Bill asked him to read the title.

"Foodborne Illnesses of Tomorrow Are Here Today," Nugent said.

Bill handed him another article and another and another, all warning of the dangers of *E. coli* in food. And all were published prior to the outbreak. In each instance he asked Nugent if he'd ever seen them.

"No I have not."

"Not that I recall."

"Not that I remember."

"No, I don't believe I have."

In all, Bill produced twenty-seven different articles from industry publications, restaurant magazines, medical journals, and newspapers that warned of *E. coli* in beef. Some of these detailed smaller *E. coli* outbreaks that preceded the Jack in the Box outbreak. And Nugent had not seen one of them.

"Does it surprise you that individuals in your quality-assurance division did not know about the *E. coli* O157:H7 bacteria?" Bill asked.

Nugent conceded that there were a lot of articles about *E. coli* in print. He had no answer for why his people had been in the dark.

Bill went back to the videotaped interview with Vieira. This time he showed a clip where Nugent was asked about Jack in the Box's meat supplier.

Vieira: Do you think that Vons knew that meat was contaminated when they sent it out?

Nugent: The testing that was done on that particular batch of meat indicated that it had high levels of *E. coli*. It is their responsibility to notify us if there's any potential hazard with a product. We were notified of those high levels of *E. coli* after the outbreak. So without notification, we couldn't take any measures to preclude it.

Bill stopped the tape. "Mr. Nugent, what were the specifications for levels of *E. coli?*"

Stearns objected, saying the question was speculative. Another lawyer objected on grounds of the question being vague and ambiguous.

Nugent waited for advice from Stearns. Then he said that prior to 1993 he hadn't known the specifications. "But," he said, "I can tell you that based upon the information that I have subsequently been given, that we had the guideline of three colonies per gram."

Next Bill handed Nugent a document that spelled out the microbiological guidelines that existed between Jack in the Box and Vons. It confirmed that three colonies of *E. coli* per gram was the standard. Anything above that was considered too high.

Then Bill handed Nugent a letter from Vons that was issued two days after the outbreak was announced. Nugent acknowledged that he was familiar with the letter.

"Okay, okay," Bill said. "And do you see the information contained under Daily Sample that indicates *E. coli* levels of 430?"

"I do, yes."

The letter also indicated that other readings showed 740 *E. coli* and 2,900 *E. coli*.

"Mr. Nugent, would you agree with me that the numbers of *E. coli*, the levels stated in the January 20, 1993, letter are above the three colonies per gram specification?"

"I do."

Bill asked Nugent if the basis of Foodmaker's lawsuit against Vons was that Vons had sent meat that had *E. coli* levels beyond the specifications.

"I'm not sure what the basis of the lawsuit is," Nugent said.

"As the president of Jack in the Box, you have *no idea* why you're suing Vons?"

Nugent was ready to explode. Stearns was, too. "I'm going to object," Stearns said impatiently, "to the form of the question being argumentative."

Bill went back to the reports showing high levels of *E. coli* in the beef patties delivered to Jack in the Box. He asked what procedure Jack in the Box had in place to insure that Vons was delivering safe meat.

Nugent said that prior to the outbreak, Jack in the Box would routinely pull food from the distribution center and subject it to testing. If problems were found, the vendor who supplied the food not meeting specifications would be notified.

Obviously, Bill said, that kind of approach hadn't worked very well.

Bill moved on to the other area he wanted to cover—the fact that Jack in the Box was not in compliance with Washington State's health code for cooking temperatures at the time of the outbreak. When he testified before the U.S. Senate weeks after the outbreak, Nugent said the company hadn't known about the rule change in Washington State. But through discovery, Bill knew otherwise. He had found a copy of the notice from the Washington State Department of Health in the files of the quality-assurance division at Jack in the Box's corporate headquarters. The date stamp on the document showed it had been received seven months prior to the outbreak.

Bill held up the notice, marked Exhibit F-65. He handed it to Nugent, who acknowledged having seen it for the first time after the outbreak.

"Do you recall how that came to your attention?" Bill asked

"Yes. It was shown to me by Ken Dunkley."

Bill handed Nugent another newspaper article, marked Exhibit F-74.

Nugent scanned it. A portion of it was highlighted in yellow. Bill asked him to read that portion aloud.

"Nugent said the company's vice president of technical services is responsible for alerting senior management to such changes, but he had not done so," Nugent read.

"And the vice president at least at the time that you spoke of was Mr. Dunkley?" Bill asked.

"Correct."

"Do you know whether or not Mr. Dunkley knew of this 155-degree cooking standard prior to the *E. coli* outbreak that brings us here today?"

"No, I don't."

"Have you ever asked Mr. Dunkley whether or not he knew of the increased cooking-temperature requirement?"

"Yes."

"And what has he told you?"

"He told me he didn't know."

The point was clear. The paper trail led right to Nugent's doorstep. The VPs who report to Nugent had either fallen down on the job or worse. Either way, Nugent had no excuse.

Bill stared at Nugent for a moment. *You're in the business, buddy, he thought to himself. You should know all this stuff, or at the very least have people in the company who know this stuff and keep you apprised.*

Before wrapping up the deposition, Bill went to the videotape one more time. He played a clip of Meredith Vieira reminding Nugent that some of the children from the outbreak will suffer the effects of their injuries for years, and she asked whether Jack in the Box was morally obliged to stay with these families over the long haul. "Maybe through their lifetime," Nugent told Vieira. "We will do that."

Bill turned off the tape and turned to Nugent. "Mr. Nugent, is that still your feeling and is that the feeling of your corporation?"

"It is stronger than ever."

"I have no further questions of this witness at this time."

43

WHAT YOU NEED

A COUPLE OF DAYS AFTER DEPOSING NUGENT, BILL WAS STILL IN SAN Diego. But Julie was encouraging him to come home right away. Suzanne had called the house looking for him, and she didn't sound well. Bill had gotten a similar report from one of the nurses assigned to the Kiner home.

But Bill still had another Jack in the Box employee to depose before returning to Seattle. Plus, he had found out that Piper was in town to meet with Jack in the Box officials. Bill didn't want to head back to Seattle before inviting Piper to dinner. Food was right up there with liquor and women on Piper's list of favorite passions, and he readily accepted. Bill suggested Rainwater's Restaurant, an upscale steakhouse.

Piper brought Stearns along. They met Bill and slid into a half-round, corner booth. Bill hoped to discuss a resolution to *Kiner* over fine wine and red meat. But Piper spent the first hour and a half telling old war stories. The night was getting on when Bill finally made his move by bringing up the fact that the depositions weren't looking very good for Jack in the Box.

Well aware of why Bill had wanted to have dinner, Piper was eager to get the *Kiner* case settled, too. In fact, he wanted all of Bill's cases out of the way. Of all the lawyers with suits against Jack in the Box, Bill was the only one with all the discovery documents. He was the only one who had connected all the dots and bothered to understand the science and the medicine. He had pieced together the paper trail that could likely convince a jury that Jack in the Box had known about the 155-degree internal temperature. The last thing Piper wanted was for other attorneys to piggyback on Bill's work.

There was one other thing Bill had that no one else had: Brianne Kiner. More than anyone, Brianne scared Piper and Jack in the Box. There were many incentives to get her case and Bill out of the way.

"Don't you think it's time we mediate these cases?" Piper asked.

Bill and Stearns were both surprised at the suggestion.

"Well, Bob, what do you have in mind?" Bill asked.

Piper started talking about the *Kiner* case and how it was "so damn *colossal.*" He seemed to relish saying that.

Bill liked the adjective, too. But he really liked what Piper said next.

"I think the time is ripe for settling the case for record money."

Stearns had to work to keep his jaw from dropping.

Bill remained steady. He didn't want to ask what Piper meant by "record money." Record money was good enough. Instead, he asked if Piper had a particular mediator in mind.

He did—retired judge Lawrence Irving. He'd been appointed to the federal bench in California by Ronald Reagan. But he'd retired in 1990 and quickly become the most highly sought-after mediator in California. He had an impeccable reputation for impartiality.

Bill wondered about the time frame.

"I think we should mediate in late January or early February," Piper said.

Bill agreed.

The back-and-forth went on for another thirty minutes or so. By the time the waiter brought the check, Bill and Piper had agreed on all the broad strokes for a mediation process. A couple of bottles of vintage wine had pushed the tab up close to a thousand dollars. Alcohol accounted for more than half of it. Broke, Bill nonetheless insisted on paying and handed over his credit card, hoping that there was some credit left on it.

Stearns had never liked Bill much . . . until now. He had a charming side to him. In that respect, he was a lot like Piper. They were two lawyers acutely focused on getting where they wanted to be at the end of the day.

Bill stood up and waited for Piper to ease out of his seat. Then he went ahead and held the door open as Piper limped outside. Before parting they shook hands.

"I'll get you what you need," Piper said.

"Thanks, Bob," Bill said before turning and nodding to Stearns.

Piper smiled wryly at Bill. "The endgame is on."

44

UNHEARD-OF

As soon as he got back to Seattle, Bill decided he wanted to set up a face-to-face meeting with Judge Irving. Before agreeing to use him as a mediator, Bill felt, it made sense to establish a rapport. Piper agreed to set something up right away.

Then Bill called attorney Rob Trentacosta in San Diego. Trentacosta had used Irving to mediate Lauren Rudolph's wrongful-death case against Jack in the Box. Bill wanted Trentacosta's take on Irving's approach. Trentacosta had nothing but good things to say about Irving, and he offered to accompany Bill when he flew down to meet the judge. Besides, Trentacosta and Rick Waite had another big case of their own that was coming up for mediation with Irving.

Everything was moving along according to plan. Then Bill's office phone rang. It was Julie. There was trouble. Suzanne had called the house again. This time she was in a state of emotional crisis, and she'd been drinking. Julie had stayed on the line with her for over an hour, attempting to calm and reassure her. But Julie was convinced Suzanne had reached the breaking point and needed help—now.

Bill asked if she knew Suzanne's whereabouts.

On a ferry, Julie reported, headed toward Bainbridge Island. The last thing Suzanne had said before hanging up was that she wanted to see Bill at his home.

Bill dropped everything and raced home in hopes of intercepting Suzanne. On the way, he placed calls from his cell phone to Brianne's case manager and Rex. The time had come, he informed them, to mobilize around Suzanne. Everyone knew what that meant. Bill had put a contingency plan in place. It was time to execute it.

Bill found Suzanne at the ferry terminal on Bainbridge Island. He took her directly to a bed-and-breakfast on the island, where Julie had reserved a room. After talking with Suzanne, he got her tucked into bed. Meantime, a detoxification-and-treatment clinic in New Mexico had been notified and was standing by. Bill had purchased Suzanne a one-way ticket out of Seattle for the following morning. He had also booked tickets for Rex and the case manager, both of whom planned to accompany Suzanne on the flight and help get her admitted to the rehab center. In the morning, Bill planned to drive Suzanne directly from the bed-and-breakfast to the airport.

The only problem with the plan was that Suzanne knew nothing about it. Bill had set the whole thing up without her input. He saw no alternative. In order for Brianne and the rest of the family to make it through the prolonged litigation process, Suzanne had to be emotionally healthy. She'd spent a year and a half helping Brianne get better. It was time for Suzanne to get some help for herself.

That night, Bill couldn't sleep. He feared Suzanne would be furious and refuse to undergo treatment once he informed her of what he had in store. The timing could not have been worse: He had just finished deposing Nugent. Piper was committed to settling the case. A mediator had been chosen. Everything was set up. Yet it was suddenly all in peril.

"What I'm about to do," he told Julie, "might get me fired."

Julie realized what was at stake. The professional and financial implications for losing the Kiner family as clients were huge. But the way Julie saw it, Brianne's best interests wouldn't be served until her mother got healthy. "It's the right thing to do," Julie told Bill. "It's the right thing to do."

Bill found Suzanne sober when he met her at the bed-and-breakfast early the following morning. A solid night's sleep in a private, cozy room had done her some good. Once Bill had her in the car, Suzanne turned to him.

"Where are you taking me?" she asked.

"The airport."

"The *airport*? What for?"

Keeping his eye on the road, Bill broke the news subtly.

Suzanne instantly started yelling at him. Then she started sobbing. The humiliation and embarrassment were hard to swallow. By the time Bill reached the airport, he wasn't sure Suzanne still wanted him to be her lawyer. But as they sat in the parking lot, she wiped her eyes and agreed to go to New Mexico. Alcohol, Bill knew, wasn't the root of the problem; it was just a symptom. He told her that he admired her courage. Most people didn't possess her strength.

After getting her checked in, he escorted her through the terminal and onto the plane. Rex and the case manager were already on board. With stewardesses and passengers looking on, Bill helped Suzanne get situated in her seat. Then he patted her on the shoulder, told her he believed in her, and walked off the plane.

The week before Christmas, Bill flew back to San Diego, where he met up with Trentacosta and Piper at a San Diego law firm where Irving maintained an office. Hollywood could not have cast someone more judicial looking than Irving. Immediately impressed, Bill could tell Irving had a strong grasp of the severity of the injuries caused by *E. coli* and HUS. Then it hit Bill: *the people with the money get to make the decisions.* In this case, the people with the money were the insurance adjusters.

Bill made a snap decision. As soon as the meeting with Irving broke up, Bill pulled Piper aside and asked him for the names and telephone numbers of the insurance adjusters at AIG and Home. Those were the two carriers whose money would be in play during the *Kiner* mediation.

Piper asked why Bill wanted the adjusters' contact information.

"Because I'm going to call them," Bill said.

Piper paused. Plaintiffs' attorneys spoke to defense attorneys, not to insurance adjusters. It was as if Bill had asked to talk directly to Jack in the Box officials. It simply wasn't done. The protocol was that lawyers talked to lawyers. In fact, Piper had never had a lawyer ask to talk to the adjusters.

Bill wasn't interested in just talking to them. He wanted to meet them.

Piper grinned and scribbled down the names on a piece of paper: Doug Brosky at AIG in New York City and the adjuster at Home in Chicago. He put their numbers under the names and handed the paper to Bill, who stepped into a private office and reached Brosky on his direct line.

Caught off guard, Brosky couldn't understand why a personal-injury lawyer from Seattle was calling him. In a thick Brooklyn accent, Brosky asked Bill what he wanted.

"I have the *Kiner* case and we're going to be mediating it in a couple of months," Bill began.

Gruff, Brosky said he knew all about the *Kiner* case. But he still couldn't figure out why Bill had called him.

"Well, it so happens that I'm going to be in New York tomorrow and I'd like to come by and meet you."

Reluctantly, Brosky agreed.

Then Bill called Chicago and talked the Home Insurance adjuster into meeting with him the following day.

Even though he was broke, Bill called back to his law office and asked the secretary to find him flights from San Diego to New York and then on to Chicago and back to Seattle. He had her charge it to his credit card. Then he called home. "Jules, I'm not coming home yet," he told Julie. "I'm going to New York."

"Why are you doing *that?*"

After he explained, she reminded him that he hadn't packed for a long trip and Christmas was only days away. Bill knew. But this was important.

"Okay," she said.

Then Bill found Trentacosta. "Rob, I'm going to New York."

Trentacosta gave Bill a weird look.

Bill told him he had just made arrangements to visit AIG before continuing on to Home's headquarters in Chicago.

Trentacosta couldn't believe it. In all his years doing personal-injury work he'd never heard of meeting directly with an adjuster. It was like going to sit down with the enemy before going to battle. It was just . . . inappropriate.

Bill smiled.

Trentacosta called Rick Waite to get his reaction. Waite found it so unheard-of he didn't know what to say either. He found it even more remarkable that the adjusters had agreed to see Bill.

Trentacosta agreed.

"That's Marler for you," Waite said.

Trentacosta hung up with Waite and grabbed Bill. "I'm going with you," Trentacosta said.

That afternoon Bill and Trentacosta boarded a flight to New York. A Long Island native, Trentacosta got a kick out of Bill's inability to stop looking up at all the tall buildings as they took a taxi to a hotel located a couple of blocks from Wall Street. Bill had never been to New York. He couldn't get over how huge it felt compared to Seattle.

The next morning they walked to AIG's headquarters, where they were greeted by Doug Brosky. Balding with wispy white hair and a perfectly trimmed beard and a ruddy complexion, Brosky stood six feet tall and wore a wool sweater. Bill extended his hand and tried to strike up a friendly conversation, but it didn't seem to work. Brosky was old school and the notion of standing face-to-face with a couple of trial lawyers was a bit too unorthodox for his liking. The meeting didn't last ten minutes.

"Well *that* went real well," Trentacosta said once they reached the street.

Bill didn't let the fact that he'd just spent a bunch of money he didn't have to fly across the country for a ten-minute encounter get to him. They had a lot of time until the flight to Chicago. Trentacosta offered to show him some sites. Bill chose Rockefeller Plaza. He'd always wanted to see the outdoor ice skating rink and the giant Christmas tree outside the NBC building.

When Bill and Trentacosta arrived at the Home office in Chicago the next day, they got another cold reception from an adjuster there— initially. A former smoker, Trentacosta observed that the adjuster kept fidgeting as Bill talked about *Kiner*.

"Would you like to go get a cigarette?" Trentacosta asked.

A few minutes later they were in a nearby coffee shop. The adjuster started chain-smoking and Bill started talking. Forty-five minutes later they were still talking. A connection had been made.

By the time they finished in Chicago, Trentacosta couldn't wait to get home, but Bill got one more idea. There was an individual in Las Vegas who had suffered serious injuries from HUS after eating a hamburger during the Jack in the Box outbreak. The injuries had been life-threatening, and the individual's lawyer was preparing to mediate with Jack in the Box and its insurers. Bill was afraid the lawyer would settle for a number that was too low, which would adversely impact the *Kiner* settlement.

Bill amended his flight plans one more time and caught a flight from Chicago to Vegas to meet with the victim's lawyer, whom he urged to delay mediation by assuring him he'd do much better by letting *Kiner* go first.

The lawyer agreed.

Months earlier, Bob Piper had tasked Bruce Clark with figuring out the fair market value of Brianne Kiner's injuries, along with some of the other serious HUS cases. With a little stronger math background, Clark could have happily gone to medical school and become a doctor. Instead he'd become a lawyer and ended up defending clients against asbestos claims and wrongful-death suits. That required him to spend more billable hours talking to physicians and reading medical journals that he did appearing in courtrooms and reading case law. Over the years he'd gotten pretty adept at calculating the cost of a person's medical injuries.

But foodborne pathogens and the potential for *E. coli* to cause lifelong medical problems put him in foreign territory. When Clark first tried digging into the research, he was fascinated by how little there was. *E. coli* O157:H7 had a pretty short history. He had to hire a pediatric nephrologist to teach him what happened when kidneys failed and what it meant to be on dialysis. He had to hire a gastroenterologist to explain what *E. coli* did to the intestines and the colon. He had to figure out the cost of a kidney transplant, as well as the other complications that could stem from *E. coli* infection. Then he had to hire an economist to project the future costs of treatments going forward.

Meantime, Clark was ready to talk numbers. Piper set up a conference call with the various insurance adjusters, since they were the ones who would ultimately cut the checks. The big question, Clark explained to the group, was what would happen to a kid like Brianne Kiner ten or fifteen or twenty years down the road. Nobody really knew. There just wasn't much precedent to look to for guidance.

This made the insurance adjusters squeamish. Nothing scares an insurer more than the inability to assess a risk.

"These kids are not going to be okay," Clark told them. "And some of these kids are apparently going to suffer kidney failure later in life. It's going to be *really* expensive."

How expensive?

"Some of these cases could be worth a few million dollars each," Clark said.

"Holy shit!" one of the adjusters boomed through the phone.

The adjusters wanted to know how many cases might fall in that range.

Clark had a simple answer: lots. And Clark hadn't even gotten to *Kiner* yet. Piper and Clark could hear the adjusters doing back-of-the-napkin calculations.

"Most renal diseases are complex," Stearns explained. "Kidney problems are not black-and-white and they are usually interrelated with other body problems."

The adjusters weren't so interested in the science. They were focused solely on the bottom line for what it was going to cost to settle with these families. And they were worried that if they overpaid Brianne Kiner, they'd establish a precedent that inflated the value of all the cases behind hers.

Piper warned them to be ready for the worst.

45

SHOW SOME BRASS

Bill and his partners met in George Kargianis's office to hash out what they'd demand from Jack in the Box to settle the *Kiner* matter. Nobody in the room had as much experience settling big cases as Kargianis. He had a reputation for being one of the shrewdest negotiators in the business. But before weighing in, Kargianis wanted to hear from his partners.

Watkins spoke up first. He thought they should get at least $3 million for *Kiner*.

Osborn immediately dismissed that figure as ridiculously low. He wanted to see them get $10 million.

"No, no, no," Bill said, insisting they should get $12 million.

A lively discussion ensued. It went on for over fifteen minutes. The only one not saying anything was Kargianis. Finally, he'd heard enough.

"Damn it!" Kargianis thundered, pounding his fist on the table. "This case is worth a hundred . . . million . . . dollars."

Everyone shut up.

Kargianis identified four areas: economic loss, compensation for Brianne's pain and suffering, Brianne's future needs in terms of medical treatment, and Brianne's projected life expectancy. "What do the experts say are the pure present and future economic costs?" he asked, facing Bill.

"They said $7 million to $8 million," Bill reported.

"Well," said Kargianis, "then the way I look at this case is that it is going to approach $10 million."

Bill shook his head in agreement.

Kargianis asked a hypothetical question. In an auto injury case with out-of-pocket costs of $10,000, would a lawyer seek a $10,000 settlement?

Everyone agreed the asking price to settle would be much higher.

Kargianis's point was clear. "You're never going to get anywhere near $10 million if you ask for $12 million," he explained. "The defense will immediately chop that in half and start hard negotiations. So you're crippling yourself in asking for something that low."

Watkins and Osborn worried that asking for $100 million would simply cause Jack in the Box to walk away. After all, the largest personal-injury settlement in the history of Washington was $10 million. They'd be seeking *ten times* that amount.

Kargianis didn't care about the current high water mark. "The *Kiner* file is compelling for a number of reasons," he explained. "First, the child suffered devastating injuries. She was injured as bad as a child could be injured."

Second, Bill had outworked everyone on this case. He had acquired incriminating documents through his dogged discovery tactics. He had mastered an understanding of the deadly *E. coli* pathogen and its medical impacts. And he had rounded up the best expert witnesses. In every respect, Bill was ready for trial.

Third, it was important to remember that Bob Piper was on the other side. He was a defense lawyer who knew how to read a demand for $100 million.

"Now dammit, let's go in and show a little brass," Kargianis said.

Bill agreed to draft a demand letter and send it over to Piper.

Piper was at his desk when the letter from Bill came over the fax machine. As soon as he read it, he recognized Kargianis's fingerprints all over the number.

"How much are they asking for?" Stearns asked.

"A hundred million dollars," Piper said, expressionless, as he tossed the letter Stearns's way.

"Holy shit!" Stearns shouted, incredulous.

"It's an opening demand. And it's meaningless," Piper said, tugging at his favorite pair of suspenders. They had silhouettes of naked women on them, similar to the ones on the mud flaps of trucks.

"But this is *outrageous*," Stearns kept on.

Piper stretched. "Don't treat it like it's your money," he said, yawning.

"But the case is worth *nowhere* near that," Stearns complained.

"A case is worth what it settles for," Piper said.

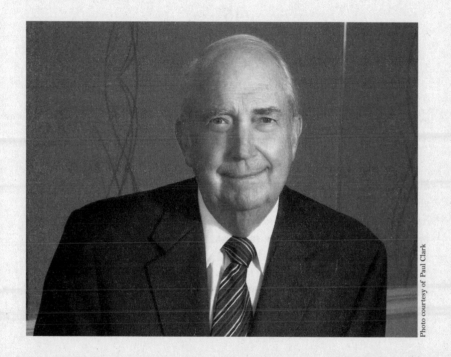

Judge Lawrence Irving mediated the high-stakes negotiations between Bill Marler and Jack in the Box.

46

FOCUSED AND FRIGHTENED

THE NEWS FROM THE KINER HOME COULD NOT HAVE BEEN BETTER. Suzanne had returned from New Mexico a changed woman. She had worked her way through a treatment program. She had gotten the upper hand on her drinking problem. Her physical stamina was up, too. Most important, her emotions were in check. Grateful to Bill for caring, she informed him that she was ready to press on.

Relieved, Bill brought her up to speed and told her to pack her bags. He had made reservations for her again. She didn't get it. He laughed and told her they were heading to a hotel in Seattle. That was where the negotiations would be held. Bill had reserved a suite there for the Kiner family.

It was early on a chilly overcast morning when Bill helped the Kiner family out of a Town Car parked in front of the massive granite and gray brick façade of the Washington Athletic Club on the corner of Sixth and Union. A couple of uniformed bellmen guided Brianne and her parents through the doors to Seattle's premier private club, leading them toward the registration desk. The facility had been chosen to host the mediation between Jack in the Box and a host of families whose children had suffered from HUS. First, Bill got the Kiners checked in to the penthouse suite on the top floor. The negotiations were expected to last a couple of days and Bill wanted Brianne and her entourage of nurses and in-home health care providers to be comfortable. In addition to the Kiners, Bill had two other client families booked at the hotel. Both had small children with HUS. Their injuries hadn't been as severe as Brianne's, but both children had undergone surgeries and had been through extensive rehab. Bill and Piper had agreed to settle those cases in conjunction with the *Kiner* case. So Bill got those two families checked into luxury suites as well.

Then Julie arrived. Bill had a room for her, too. A lot was riding on what would transpire over the next forty-eight hours. To Julie the negotiations represented a culmination of everything Bill had done during the previous two years working on the Jack in the Box outbreak. Whatever happened, she wanted to be there to support him. He'd come a long way from being fired and unable to land a job. With a fresh haircut and a brand new pair of stylish glasses with circular lenses, Bill looked a lot like Bruce Willis in *The Bonfire of the Vanities*. Only Bill was for real. And he was hers. She kissed him on the lips and wished him luck.

Bill took the elevator down to the floor where the mediation was scheduled to take place. He immediately spotted Piper, seated like a sentinel in an easy chair parked at the entrance to the mediation room. He was wearing wrinkled trousers and his trademark suspenders and sports coat over a white shirt and tie. His gut seemed larger than ever. No one was getting in that room without passing Piper and his gaze.

Bill nodded at him, then took a deep breath and entered the room. More than twenty-five trial lawyers and a dozen insurance adjusters were milling around. Some of the lawyers had cases to mediate. Others were just there to watch the *Kiner* mediation. All eyes were on Bill, who looked way too young to be the center of attention.

"Hey, Bill."

Bill turned around to see who had called his name. It was AIG's adjuster Doug Brosky.

"How are you?" Brosky asked.

Bill smiled and extended his hand. "Hi, Doug, good to see you."

In a roomful of lawyers, Bill was the only one Brosky knew. The same was true for the adjuster from Home Insurance. The fact that they had met Bill a few weeks earlier somehow made them feel as though Bill were a familiar commodity. That brand of retail politics—building those interpersonal relationships that minimize the disdain in an adversarial process—was what Bill had mastered as a city councilman during his college days. None of these adjusters had ever struck up a friendly rapport with an opposing personal-injury lawyer. The collegial greeting took the edge off.

Judge Irving brought the group to order and outlined the procedures for the mediation. He acknowledged the presence of many lawyers and the fact that there were many cases to mediate. But the first cases on the docket were the three belonging to Bill Marler. This was Jack in the Box's preference. Not only did Bill have the biggest cases, but unknown to the other lawyers, he was also the only lawyer in the building with all the embarrassing internal documents from the fast-food chain. There was a lot of incentive to get rid of Bill's cases first.

To begin, Irving had Bill and the Jack in the Box legal team go into separate rooms. The opening offer from the insurance companies was $2 million to settle *Kiner*. The entire first day was chewed up trying to get Jack in the Box to come up and Marler to come down.

On the second day, the insurance companies wanted to continue discussing *Kiner*, but Bill thought it made more sense to focus on his other two cases. The two sides weren't as far apart on those numbers.

"Judge, I think we're really close on these other cases," Bill told Irving. "But we're not close on *Kiner*."

Irving agreed.

Bill explained that he thought the insurers would like to see all three cases settled as a group. He also felt the insurers would pay more to settle *Kiner* if they knew all three cases could get disposed of at once.

"I think you're right," Irving said.

"So I'd like to keep going on the two that we're close on," Bill said.

Irving felt that was fine. But it would help him to know Bill's bottom line on the Kiner case. "What do you think the *Kiner* case should settle for?" Irving asked.

"Nineteen million," Bill said.

Irving stared at him.

"Nineteen million," Bill repeated softly.

"I don't have any indication what they'll pay," Irving said, clearly shocked by the number.

The two sides agreed to set *Kiner* aside and focus on Bill's other two cases. Over the next six hours, Irving went back and forth with them on numbers and terms. Late in the afternoon of the second day, Irving entered Bill's suite and reported that the other side was prepared to settle Bill's first two cases for $3.5 million and $4.5 million, respectively. Bill and Kargianis had evaluated those cases at around $3 million each.

Bill thought for a moment. Nobody knew it, but Bill and Julie had exhausted their line of credit and maxed out their credit cards. They were three months behind on their mortgage payment. Due to Bill's work, the firm was doing slightly better—it was finally back to a break-even point. But even there Bill had racked up a lot of expenses with travel and expert witnesses in preparation for the mediation. Bill had successfully held the firm and his family together, all along looking to the outside world as if things were more than fine. But he was holding the finances together with a shoestring and he'd been working these *E. coli* cases for almost two years. It was imperative that he pull in some revenue.

"I'll settle the first two," Bill told Irving.

Irving left the room to tell the insurance adjusters that they had a deal on the first two cases. Then it sank in: he had just settled $8 million worth of cases. It was hard to imagine.

Thirty minutes later Irving returned and confirmed the settlement of the first two cases.

Bill tried to remain cool. But he was tempted to pinch himself. Eight million dollars!

"Now," Irving said, "I have an offer for you on Kiner."

Bill's heart raced. "What is it?"

"Twelve million."

Bill did some quick math in his head: *$8 million for the first two cases plus $12 million for Kiner equals $20 million. Insurance guys like nice round numbers.*

"That's not enough," Bill said.

Irving asked if Bill wanted to make a counteroffer.

"Sixteen million," he said.

While waiting to hear back from Irving, Bill stepped out for some fresh air. He ran into Piper in the lobby. "We're not going to pay any more money than $12 million," he said gruffly.

"Then you're not going to settle the *Kiner* case," Bill said.

Piper smiled and immediately changed the subject. He began talking about the other lawyers waiting with cases behind Bill.

The Kiners were getting antsy. They'd been on pins and needles for two days. Staying in the presidential suite was nice. But they were eager—very eager—to settle and move on. Bill was updating Suzanne and Rex when there was a knock on the door. It was Judge Irving. Bill excused himself and stepped out into the hallway with him.

"Bill, they will pay $14 million," he said. "But they will not pay a penny more."

Bill needed a minute to think. Just a little while earlier Piper had assured him they were topped out at $12 million, and they'd just come up to $14 million. That was $4 million more than the largest personal-injury settlement in state history. George Kargianis was right when he said that to get what you want you need to show some brass. Bill had made up his mind.

"You're Honor, I'm not going to settle it for $14 million," Bill told Irving.

Floored, Irving stared at him in silence.

"I'm not going to settle it," Bill repeated, feeling weak in the knees. Then he turned and headed toward the door to the Kiners' room.

"Bill," Irving called out.

He turned and looked at Irving.

"Can I talk to you for a moment?" Irving asked. His tone was more like, *Now young man, you listen to me.*

"Sure," Bill said, walking back to him.

"Bill, this is an *awful* lot of money."

Bill shook his head.

"Look, I trust you," Irving said. "But I want to make sure your clients are on board . . . because *$14 million* is an awful lot of money."

"I know, Your Honor. But I'm not going to take it."

"You're not going to take it?" Irving asked.

"No."

"Well, what's your number?"

"What I told you earlier: $16 million."

Irving folded his arms and turned his head from side to side. "They're not going to pay it."

Bill shrugged his shoulders and turned up his hands.

"If I can get them to fifteen, would you take it?" Irving asked.

"No. It's got to be sixteen."

Irving dropped his chin and nodded. It was the end of the day and he was exhausted. "Well," he said, looking up with a smile. "You settled $8 million worth of cases today. But you're not going to settle *Kiner*." He turned and walked off.

The way Bill looked at it settling $8 million worth of cases was more than most lawyers did in a career. So the pressure was off. His and Julie's financial worries were behind them and the firm was headed for the black. It gave him the confidence to push the envelope on *Kiner*. No one, not even Kargianis or Brad Keller or any other top lawyer in Seattle had negotiated a personal-injury case in the $15 million range. Bill was in no-man's land . . . and he felt at home.

Suzanne and Rex were waiting for him when he returned to their suite.

"What'd he say?" Suzanne asked enthusiastically.

Bill led Suzanne and Rex into a private room.

"They offered $14 million . . ." he began.

Suzanne put her hand over her mouth.

". . . and I turned them down."

Suzanne squeezed her lips. Rex tried to stay poised. They'd given Bill full authority to say yes or no to a deal. But they couldn't grasp turning down $14 million. It was as if they'd had the wind knocked out of them.

"But I'm convinced they will pay more," Bill added. "I ask you to trust me that that will happen."

Bruce Clark, Denis Stearns, and Bob Piper were huddled in their meeting room with all the insurance adjusters. No one could get over Bill Marler's audacity.

"Where does a young, inexperienced guy like that get off being so ballsy?" one of them remarked.

"Greedy bastard's what he is," another adjuster said.

To the insurers, paying anyone over $10 million was insane.

"Nobody could spend that much money in their lifetime," one of the adjusters insisted.

Clark said little. He actually admired Bill's chutzpa. The guy had outhustled everyone and now he was sitting in the driver's seat. More power to him.

But Piper had heard enough. He wasn't about to let the *Kiner* negotiations get strung out any further. These adjusters needed a reality check.

"You're money's f——n' gone!" Piper told them. "This thing is going off the rails. And once it goes off the rails, no one will be able to get it back."

Deep down, everyone knew what Piper was getting at. If a deal wasn't struck with Marler, the *Kiner* case would end up going to trial. That would touch off a chain reaction of bad events for Jack in the Box and its insurers. First, all the other victims that were in line to settle would have second thoughts. Their lawyers would advise them to pull back in order to see what *Kiner* got from a jury. Next, buckets of money would be spent trying the case. Then it would all be in the hands of a Seattle jury. The last thing Jack in the Box wanted was for a few Seattle mothers on a jury to be deciding how much Brianne Kiner deserved for her injuries. Whatever amount came out of that process would establish a new benchmark for all the other kids with less serious injuries.

Piper let the adjusters stew in all this while he placed a call to San Diego. He spelled out his position in terms that Jack Goodall would understand. In front of a jury in King County the sky would be the limit for Brianne Kiner. And if they let Bill Marler ring that bell, then everyone else was going to line up at the trough and want extra money because of some perceived huge bonus that went to the Kiners as a result of taking the insurers to the mat. Or, Piper explained, Foodmaker and its insurers could make a public demonstration that they were willing to be more than fair.

The ball was in Jack in the Box's court.

———————

Bill went back to his room to call his law partners. They'd been waiting anxiously for an update. They gathered around a speaker phone to get the news.

"I just want to let you know that I settled the first two cases for a total of $8 million," Bill said.

"Yeah!" they shouted.

"And," he said, talking over them, "and—"

They quieted down.

". . . they offered $14 million on *Kiner*."

"YEAHHHH!" they screamed.

Bill had to pull the phone back from his ear. He waited for them to calm down.

"And I turned them down," he said.

It was if the phone had gone dead. No sound. Nothing.

"You *what?*" Kargianis finally said.

"I think they'll pay more," Bill said.

If Bill's hunch was wrong, he and his firm were headed to trial. That could take another couple of years to resolve.

Bill knew that better than anyone.

Julie entered the room as Bill hung up the phone. He looked as if he'd just run a marathon. When Bill removed his suit coat, his shirt clung to his skin with perspiration.

"So how did it go today?" she asked.

He told her that he's settled his first two cases for $8 million. She listened patiently as he rehearsed the negotiation steps and how pleased he was with the outcome.

"So what's going on with the Kiners?" she asked.

He told her that he had rejected Jack in the Box's offer to settle for $14 million.

She raised her eyebrows and pushed her tongue up against the inside of her top lip.

He widened his eyes and puffed up his cheeks.

"O-o-o-kay," she said slowly.

Bill wasn't sure what would happen next. But whatever it was, he was sure it wouldn't happen before morning.

"Honey," he said, "you might as well go home. I've got a few loose ends to tie up here. I'll meet you at the house later tonight."

47

THE MAGNETIC MOMENT

Exhausted, Bill wasn't quite ready to call it a night. He had an idea. He took the elevator down to the second floor and headed to the suite reserved by Piper and the adjusters. He knocked on the door and entered without waiting for a response.

"Who is it?" someone shouted.

By then Bill was inside and upon them.

"Hey guys," he said, as if they were all buddies.

No one knew how to react. Only the mediator was allowed in the opposing side's room. This was a clear violation of mediation decorum.

"What the hell do *you* want?" one of the adjusters finally said.

Bill smiled. "No hard feelings," he said, extending his hand, as he made his way around the table. "I know you're all working hard on this and I just wanted to say that I appreciate it. And I'd like to buy all you guys a drink."

The insurance adjusters and Stearns and Clark didn't know what to say. They were in the thick of a heated mediation and adversaries weren't supposed to raise a glass together.

But Piper thought that hitting the hotel bar was a damn good idea. He got up and led the way.

The wide planks on the wooden floor looked as if they were right out of an old western saloon. Wall sconces lit the place. A couple of silver beer steins bookended the counter. They pulled two tables together before plopping down in burgundy leather chairs with wooden armrests. Bill told the waiter the drinks were on him. Piper ordered his favorite—vodka on the rocks.

As soon as the drinks arrived, one of the adjusters started in on Bill.

"You greedy bastard," he said, a cigarette in one hand and a drink in the other. "Fourteen million is a lotta damn money. It's *A LOTTA* damn money!"

Bill sipped his whiskey and said nothing.

"Shit, you could structure it, fa God's sake," the adjuster continued.

The other agents nodded in agreement, their glasses already drained.

Bill kept his composure as the adjuster continued.

Suddenly Bill's cell phone rang. Assuming it was Julie, he took the call.

"Hey, honey, what's up?"

"Ah, Bill, it's Judge Irving."

"Oh," Bill said, cupping his mouth and stumbling as he tried to get away from the table. The adjuster was still swearing at him.

"Hello, Your Honor."

Irving could hardly hear him over all the background commotion. "Bill, *where* are you?"

"I'm in the bar with all the insurance guys."

"Can you get out in the hallway for a second?"

"Yeah, sure." He turned to Piper and the others. "It's the wife. I'll be right back guys."

Bill scurried to a quiet place in the lobby.

"Is there a number between 15 and 16 that you will take?" Irving asked.

Bill felt an adrenaline rush. "It's got to be 16," Bill said.

"I am recommending," Irving said deliberately and forcefully, "that you take $15.6 million."

Bill paused. His true target all along had been $12 million. So he'd been playing with the house's money all day. But in his mind it was justified—Brianne deserved it. She'd been through hell. And the bigger the penalty, the more the food industry would stand up and take notice that it needed to change its ways.

Irving waited for Bill's answer. "You will not get any more money," he said, emphatically, pointing out that he had spoken to Jack Goodall directly. The Foodmaker CEO had pledged to press the insurance companies to give a little more. "So I am recommending you take it, Bill. Right now. Fifteen point six million. I'm asking and suggesting you take it."

In negotiations there's a moment when the magnets on the two sides are so close you know they will snap together. Bill sensed that moment had arrived.

"I'll settle for 15.6," he told Irving.

Irving congratulated him.

"So it's done?" Bill asked.

"Not quite," Irving said, explaining that the insurers still had to sign on. But Goodall had a gun to their heads. He expected the insurers to give into Foodmaker's wishes rather than risk a greater judgment if the case went to trial.

"Bill, listen, you can't tell anybody else that you've got the case settled until I confirm it in the morning," Irving said. "But you've got a deal."

Bill felt like a new man. Between *Kiner* and the other two cases, he'd settled $23.6 million worth of cases in one day. That was more than most lawyers did in a career. He strolled back into the bar. The insurer with the cigarette started in on him again. "You're one greedy bastard, Marler," he said.

Bill smiled and signaled the bartender to send another round over—on him. Then he downed one more whiskey, said goodnight, paid the tab, and headed home to Julie. It was going to be a night of little sleep. He planned to tell her it was finally time to look for a house on Bainbridge Island.

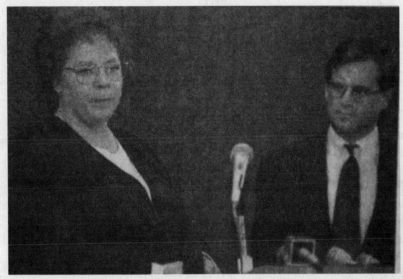

Suzanne Kiner (L), speaking to the media after Bill Marler (R), negotiated a record-breaking settlement for Brianne Kiner.

48

ENOUGH MONEY TO GO AROUND

"$15.6 MILLION *E. COLI* CASE SETTLEMENT." THE HEADLINE in the *Seattle Times* had the whole city talking, especially those standing around the water coolers at law firms. The newspaper pointed out that the agreement between Jack in the Box and Brianne Kiner represented the largest personal-injury award in state history. "In the context of what she went through, this is a very fair settlement," Bill told the paper. "I think the settlement is a recognition on the part of Foodmaker, Inc., that they cannot with impunity ignore food-safety regulations."

Even the lawyers at Bob Piper's firm couldn't grasp the size of the award.

"That $15.6 million is what Brianne will get over her lifetime through an annuity, right?" one lawyer asked Bruce Clark. "That's not $15.6 million in present-day cash value?"

"No," Clark said, grinning. "That's the present value of the settlement."

"Holy shit!" the lawyer said, shaking his head.

"Holy shit is right," Clark said, laughing raucously. "It's a colossal sum."

But Piper got what he wanted. With Kiner and Marler out of the way, Jack in the Box was in position to rapidly start extinguishing the hundreds of other claims. A ceiling had been established. And no one else was going to get near it.

Bill was suddenly a very popular guy. News of his record settlement award for Brianne Kiner had reached *USA Today*. Bill was getting calls of congratulations from people he hadn't talked to in years.

The first thing Bill did was help get Brianne enrolled in a top-notch institution in New Mexico that offered schooling and therapy. Then he turned his attention to dividing up the legal fees. The first $1.6 million of *Kiner*'s settlement was dedicated to medical expenses. Bill took no fee from that portion. On the remaining $14 million he cut his fee from the standard 33 percent to 20 percent, which amounted to $2.8 million. Half of that went to Keller Rohrback under the mediation agreement he'd reached with them a year earlier. That left $1.4 million, of which 60 percent went to Bill's three law partners to split amongst themselves, leaving Bill $560,000. It would have been easy to stew over the $2.2 million he paid out to other lawyers who did virtually no work on the *Kiner* case, but instead of looking back, Bill looked ahead. He had enough to pay cash for the dream home that Julie had picked out along the beachfront of Bainbridge Island.

Meantime, Bill wanted to do something for the group that's always forgotten: the office staff. He knew better than anyone how much the paralegals and secretaries had worked on the *Kiner* case. Frankly, they'd done way more work than Bill's law partners. In his mind they deserved a bonus.

Bill told his partners he wanted to set aside a hundred thousand dollars from their combined fee and divide it up amongst the office staff.

He faced resistance.

"C'mon you guys," Bill said. "These people all worked hard."

The partners countered that the staff had also drawn a weekly salary for the past two years while the partners had given up their salaries because of the firm's financial difficulties.

"No, no," Bill said. "We gotta do it."

To Bill it wasn't a hard sacrifice. Besides, there were more fees coming in from the other two cases Bill had settled at the Washington Athletic Club. So there was plenty of money to go around. But the more Bill pushed, the harder his partners pushed back. They simply weren't going to do it.

Disgusted, Bill stormed out. "You should be happy this whole damn thing happened," he shouted. "You should give the staff the money and go out and buy me a damn gold Rolex watch."

Two days later Mike Watkins bought Bill a gold Rolex. And the office staff got their hundred thousand dollars' worth of bonuses.

After the final settlement checks arrived from the insurance companies, Bill called Keller Rohrback and let the firm know he'd be dropping off a certified check in accordance with their agreement.

It felt a little strange to step off the elevator into the lobby of his old law firm. The last time he'd done that was the night he'd cleaned out his office over two years earlier. This time he was there to hand over a check in excess of $2 million. He approached the reception desk.

"Hi, Bill," the receptionist said, smiling. She had always liked Bill. "Go ahead back. Kirk is in his office."

Kirk Portman had signed the mediation agreement between Bill and the firm. He was eager to see Bill. He grinned as Bill entered his office. Bill reached into his suit jacket pocket and removed an envelope and pushed it across Portman's desk.

Portman removed the check, glanced at it and smiled. It's not every day that someone hands you a check for $2 million.

They chatted collegially for a few minutes.

"You should come back to work here," Portman joked.

Bill laughed. "I don't think so."

They shook hands and Bill left. He never heard from Sarko or Pence.

Bob Nugent wanted to kiss the feet of Paul Carter, the director on Jack in the Box's board who had convinced the company to raise its liability coverage from $40 million to $100 million back in 1992. In the end, it took over $98 million in insurance to extinguish all the damage claims from the *E. coli* outbreak. Without Carter, the company wouldn't have survived.

Nugent, however, still had a tough call to make. After suffering huge losses in 1993 and 1994, Jack in the Box saw sales spike up in the first quarter of 1995. The uptick was the result of a new television ad campaign featuring a character named Jack the CEO, who wore a clown head. The remarkably catchy ad started running in January 1995 and it announced that the restaurant chain's signature burger—the Jumbo Jack—was now on sale for ninety-nine cents. Sales took off like a rocket. But at the end of March the company stopped discounting the

Jumbo Jack and profits fell back to negative levels. The company had burned through all its cash reserves and Nugent figured bankruptcy was inevitable. There was no way Jack in the Box could survive a third year of huge losses.

Then some of the marketing team made a suggestion to Nugent: since the ninety-nine-cent Jumbo Jack had driven sales in the first quarter of 1995, why not go back to that and maintain that rock-bottom price indefinitely? With nothing to lose, Nugent went for it. Within a year the company returned to profitability.

Meantime, Dave Theno's food safety system got implemented throughout the company's nearly 1,200 restaurants. Various aspects of the plan were picked up by the federal government and incorporated into the USDA's new meat-inspection regulations. The company's board of directors made Theno an executive officer of the corporation.

At the end of 1995, Bill went to the office over the Christmas holiday. It was a Monday morning and there was a message from Piper on his voice mail, complaining about something. "Call me," Piper growled.

Since settling the *Kiner* case, Bill had picked up many new clients from the outbreak who had been referred to him by other lawyers. Bill figured that was what Piper wanted to talk about. He got Piper's secretary on the phone and asked to speak with Piper.

Her voice melted into tears. "He died yesterday," she said.

"What?"

Stunned, Bill hung up the phone. Suddenly, that last voice mail felt like a voice from the grave.

On January 6, 1996, Piper's wake was held at an Irish restaurant and bar in Seattle. The place was packed with lawyers, many of whom had been his adversaries over the years. Bill and Julie attended together. Piper's ashes were present, alongside a vodka martini. The martini was half empty.

49

IT'S IN JUICE, TOO

A Few Months Later

BILL WAS IN HIS LAW OFFICE WHEN A REPORTER FROM THE ASSOCIATED Press called. The CDC had traced an *E. coli* outbreak to apple juice made by Odwalla, a California company. At the time, virtually all juice companies, from Tropicana to Nantucket Nectars, pasteurized their juice, a process that kills bacteria with extreme heat. But Odwalla made a name for itself by producing freshly squeezed, unpasteurized juices and smoothies. The approach caught on quickly among consumers seeking better nutrition from fresh fruits and vegetables. But now Odwalla was being blamed for a rash of illnesses traced to bad apples. The idea that *E. coli* could land in fresh produce had people scared. The reporter wanted Bill's reaction.

The next day he was quoted in the AP story and his phone started ringing. The first call came from a lawyer in Washington, DC. He represented a couple in Colorado whose child was dying from *E. coli* complications stemming from Odwalla juice. The attorney admitted knowing nothing about foodborne illness and asked Bill if he'd assist the family. The next call came from a couple in Seattle. Both parents worked for Microsoft. They had purchased juice for their child at a Seattle-area Starbucks. Now their child was hospitalized. They wanted Bill's help. Then Bill got a call from a state senator in Chicago. His five-year-old granddaughter had recently visited Seattle with her mother. Before returning home, they stopped at a Starbucks en route to the airport. The mother got a latte and the daughter got Odwalla apple juice. Four days later she was on kidney dialysis at a Chicago-area hospital. The senator wanted to fly out to Seattle to meet with Bill in hopes that he'd take the family's case.

The wheels in Bill's mind started turning. If *E. coli* had found its way into apples, did that mean that all fresh produce was potentially vulnerable to *E. coli* contamination? If so, this food bug was going to become the number one hazard to America's food system.

Something else occurred to him. The families that he was getting calls from in the Odwalla outbreak were different than the ones he had represented in the Jack in the Box outbreak. Odwalla was a pricy product marketed to health-conscious consumers. The parents who could afford it were the same ones who largely avoided feeding their kids fast food because of health concerns. These were parents who were accustomed to spending more in order to insure that their kids were eating the most wholesome foods.

Following the Jack in the Box *case, Bill Marler represented scores of children sickened during an* E. coli *outbreak linked to apple juice.*

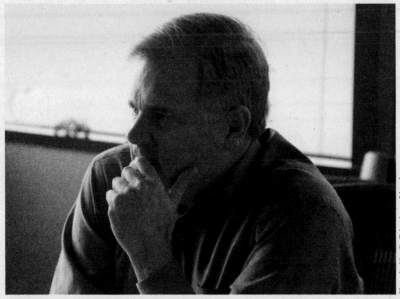

Photo by Natalie Fobes/www.fobesphoto.com

Bill said yes to the lawyer in DC and to the couple from Microsoft and to the politician in Chicago. But he knew he needed help. Odwalla had retained one of the largest defense firms in San Francisco. Plus, he wouldn't be taking on just Odwalla: Starbucks was the retailer. There was no way he could sue Odwalla and Starbucks without help—a lot of help.

But none of the partners in his law office had really worked on the *Jack in the Box* case. They knew very little about *E. coli*. He needed someone with experience, or a couple of people with experience.

Then he got an idea. When it came to foodborne illness litigation, there were only two lawyers who had as much experience as he did: Denis Stearns and Bruce Clark. Better still, they knew all the tactics and strategies from the perspective of a food company whose product had made children sick with *E. coli*. They'd spent three years in the trenches defending Jack in the Box. They handled everything: discovery, expert witnesses, insurance payouts—you name it.

Bill picked up the phone and called Stearns. "Hey, Denis, this is Marler."

Stearns was surprised.

"Hey, would you have any interest in coming on board with me to take on Odwalla?"

EPILOGUE

BILL MARLER ENDED UP REPRESENTING MOST OF THE CHILDREN WHO
were seriously injured in the Odwalla *E. coli* outbreak. Denis Stearns
agreed to join him and handled the discovery process in the litigation
against the juice maker. Most of these claims were settled by Bill in 1998
for a reported $15 million.

After the Odwalla case, Bill left Kargianis, Watkins & Marler and
started his own firm with Denis Stearns.* They persuaded Bruce Clark
to join them in the formation of Marler Clark LLP, the nation's first
personal-injury firm dedicated to litigating foodborne illness and bacterial
outbreaks. Over the past fifteen years, the firm has won more than $600
million in settlements and verdicts on behalf of children made ill by
invisible viruses, bacteria, parasites, and toxins that increasingly show up
in food that's been stamped "safe" by the USDA and FDA. Bill has been
approached to run for public office again, the Senate or Congress. He, to
Julie's pleasure, has declined.

Now fifty-three years old, Bill is the number one foodborne illness
litigator in the world. But he's more than that. He's a food safety activist,
a politician, and a media virtuoso who blogs and tweets and has videos
on YouTube. He owns thirty websites dedicated to food and its safety.
And he is the founder of *Food Safety News*, the nation's first online daily
newspaper dedicated to covering the issues surrounding food safety that
most newspapers ignore. He is a sought after speaker throughout the

---

*Osborn had left the firm after the Kiner settlement.

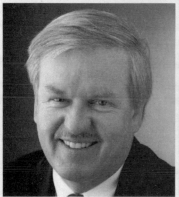
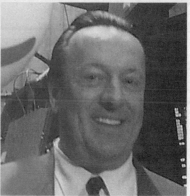
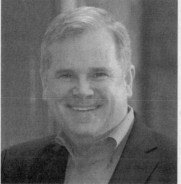
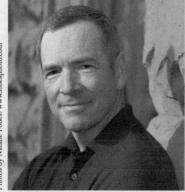
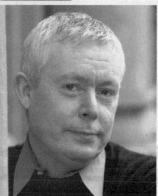

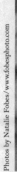

Left to right: Dave Theno, Bob Nugent,
Bill Marler,
Bruce Clark, Denis Stearns

world where he frequently tells the food industry "why it is a bad idea to poison your customers."

The food industry thinks of Bill as Marler the SOB, albeit a respected one. That's because he does things most lawyers wouldn't dare. Once he took along his digital camera after getting a court order to inspect the peanut factory responsible for a *Salmonella* outbreak that led to the biggest food recall in U.S. history. He later posted on his blog the pictures he took of rodent feces, challenging the CEO of the peanut company to come clean and the government to put the CEO in jail. Another time he interrogated the CEO of a fast-food chain by showing him graphic pictures of a comatose nine-year-old girl whose large intestine had to be removed after being ravaged by an *E. coli*–tainted hamburger.

Like any self-made man, Bill Marler has his own style. Friends and foes alike call it "the Marler Way."

After the settlement, Suzanne Kiner continued to be a powerful advocate for changes to our nation's food safety laws. Today she lives alone in Mukilteo, Washington, where she maintains a private life. Her daughter Brianne turned twenty-seven in 2011. Brianne's immune system remains compromised. She has high blood pressure, and she does not have the stamina to work an eight-hour day.

But she owns her own home, has a great circle of friends, and appreciates every new day. For a period of time she worked part-time at Bill Marler's law firm. In 2010 she started taking cooking classes at a culinary school in the Seattle area. She's found that she loves working with food. Her mother summed it up this way: "Brianne is the happiest I've seen her since Christmas of 1992." And although a bit worn, the teddy bear with the blue bowtie is still with her.

Jack in the Box survived the outbreak and eventually returned to profitability in 1996. The company has been profitable every year since. In fiscal year 2010, net earnings were $70.2 million. And with over 2,200 restaurants now in operation, Jack in the Box ranks fifth overall in nationwide sales for hamburger chains, behind McDonald's, Burger King, Wendy's, and Sonic. Bob Nugent was at the helm for this remarkable recovery. He retired as the company's CEO on October 2, 2005. Today he lives a low-profile life with his wife, outside San Diego.

"I've been working for over fifty years," he told me. "It's lovely to get up and have nothing to do."

Dave Theno deserves equal credit for Jack in the Box's revival. He left the company in October 2008 and went into retirement. "But I flunked retirement 101," he told me. He and his wife launched Gray Dog Partners, Inc., a food-technology and food safety consulting firm. Ken Dunkley eventually left Jack in the Box, too. But not before creating many new products that are now standard in the fast-food industry, including the grilled sourdough burger and the fajita pita. He also created Quick Stuff, Jack in the Box's proprietary convenience store concept, which combines mini-restaurants with a convenience store and branded gasoline stations operated by the fast-food chain. After leaving Jack in the Box, Dunkley formed a California-based consulting firm called Quick Foods Consulting in 2005. He remains there today.

In California, no mother did more to change food safety laws than Roni Austin. She teamed up with Dave Theno and together they lobbied relentlessly for reforming the state's laws on food safety. In 1997 Roni testified before the California State Assembly. Later that year the state passed the Lauren Beth Rudolph Food Safety Act. Roni was also on hand at the White House on July 6, 1996, when President Bill Clinton announced new USDA regulations adopting HACCP, essentially standardizing the inspection procedures implemented by Jack in the Box. Still, Roni says, the void left by Lauren's absence will never heal.

———————

Major outbreaks continue to occur, many of them involving *E. coli*. In 2006 an *E. coli* outbreak linked to Taco Bell restaurants swept through the Northeast. New York and New Jersey were the hardest hit. Lettuce was the culprit. The same year, fresh spinach infected more than 200 people in 26 states with *E. coli*. Five people died. Then, in 2007 the FDA advised consumers not to eat ConAgra's Peter Pan brand of peanut butter after 425 people in 44 states were infected with *Salmonella*. Viruses, bacteria, parasites, and toxins have made their way into virtually every food product on the market.

All of this has kept Marler on the forefront of food-safety matters. In addition to representing clients in all of these major outbreaks, he took on the case of nineteen-year-old dancer Stephanie Smith, who was sickened by an *E. coli*–tainted hamburger that left her brain damaged and paralyzed in 2007. In 2009, *New York Times* writer Michael Moss won a Pulitzer Prize for his coverage of Smith's case, which was settled by Cargill in 2010 for an amount "to take care of her for life."

In 2009, Linda Rivera, a fifty-seven-year-old mother of six from Nevada, was stricken with what Dr. Siegler described as "the severest multi-organ (bowel, kidney, brain, lung, gall bladder, and pancreas) case of *E. coli* mediated HUS I have seen in my extensive experience." Rivera's story hit the front page of the *Washington Post* and became an impetus for moving the FDA Food Safety Modernization Act through Congress.

Marler was a major force behind getting the landmark legislation signed into law by President Obama in 2011. It was just one aspect of Marler's overall effort to go well beyond simply litigating cases. In 1999 he emerged as the most outspoken advocate for banning the sale of raw milk. He successfully lobbied California governor Arnold Schwarzenegger to veto a 1999 bill that would have lessened standards for raw-milk safety. He also lobbied Wisconsin governor Jim Doyle to prohibit the sale of unpasteurized milk in that state. At the same time, Marler convinced Whole Foods to discontinue the sale of raw milk as of March 2010.

Meantime, six new strains of *E. coli*—known as non-O157s—have surfaced. They are just as lethal as the strain in the Jack in the Box outbreak. The CDC estimates that these strains poison thirty-seven thousand people each year and kill nearly thirty. In 2007, Marler had a thirteen-year-old client who died from eating food contaminated with one of these unregulated strains. That prompted Bill to commission IEH Laboratories & Consulting Group to conduct a five-hundred-thousand-dollar private study. The group analyzed five thousand samples of meat randomly purchased from grocery stores throughout the U.S. One percent of the store-bought meat was contaminated with these non-O157 strains of *E. coli*.

That may not sound like much, but it is: Each year Americans consume billions of pounds of ground beef. If 1 percent is contaminated with these unregulated strains of *E. coli*, millions of pounds of poisonous meat are being eaten annually. During the summer of 2010, Marler turned his test results over to the USDA. The meat industry countered with a letter arguing that no reported outbreaks in the U.S. had been directly linked to beef products. Days later, the USDA announced that Cargill Meat Solutions, one of the biggest beef suppliers in the U.S., had recalled roughly 8,500 pounds of ground beef products that may have been contaminated with *E. coli* O26, one of the non-O157 strains. The announcement came after the CDC reported two patients in Maine and one in New York had contracted a rare strain of *E. coli* after consuming beef. The only reason the CDC found out about these three people was that their stool cultures happened to have been analyzed at one of the few labs in the U.S. that tests for non-O157 strains.

To get the USDA to stop dragging its feet on implementing testing procedures for the non-O157 strains, Marler threatened to sue the agency in 2011. A few months later in 2011 a massive outbreak tied to a non-O157 strain of *E. coli* in imported fenugreek seeds from Egypt swept across Europe. More than four thousand people were sickened and fifty people died. On September 13, 2011, the federal government finally outlawed such strains of *E. coli* in the American food supply.

Bill has not shied away from controversy. In 2012 the beef industry was turned upside down when consumers—and then restaurants and grocery stores— stopped purchasing an additive to hamburger that the industry called "Lean Finely Textured Beef" (or LFTB) but that had taken on the name "Pink Slime" in the media. Beef Products Inc., the maker of LFTB quickly shuttered three of its four plants and within months sued ABC News, several reporters and producers, and two former USDA employees for $1.2 billion. Bill is defending the two retired USDA workers pro bono.

"What I'm doing with my life is exactly what I wanted to do with my life," Marler told me after I finished writing *Poisoned*. We were in his corner office during a rare moment of reflection in his otherwise bullet-fast life. A twenty-page client case list rested on the pine table beside him. It's a spreadsheet listing the names of his firm's clients, the specific foodborne illness outbreak that made each of them sick, the name of the illness, the company responsible, and the cost of the damages. It's the first thing Marler looks at each morning. At any given time, there are close to one thousand clients on the list and upward of $100 million in pending damage awards. It's easy to see that food poisoning outbreaks have become big business and his firm will soon eclipse $1 billion in settlements and verdicts from the industrial food processors responsible for the problem.

He steps back from the window. The time for reflection has passed. His iPhone is vibrating—it's the *New York Times*. The in-box on the screen of his razor-thin iMac is filling up with emails reporting the latest outbreak. His signature is needed on a demand letter. A junior associate needs his ear on a case. A defense lawyer from a beef producer is on line one wanting to negotiate. And Marler's due to post something on one of his food poison blogs.

But I have one last question.

"When you were a teenager, what did you want to be?"

"I always knew," he said, clearing his throat, "even when I was a little kid that I was going to do something important. I can't tell you there was a specific moment that I felt that way. I just always knew."

ACKNOWLEDGMENTS

For a couple of years my wife, Lydia, kept telling me to write a book on the food industry. I resisted, saying guys like Michael Pollan and Eric Schlosser did that. I write nonfiction stories, usually ones built around legal disputes. So I passed.

Meantime, Lydia revolutionized the way our family eats. One week she cleaned out our cupboards and refrigerator, getting rid of everything from brand-name cereal to frozen meat to staple products like butter, flour, and sugar. Even the salt and pepper went. She restocked our kitchen with organic foods bought primarily from local farmers' markets. We also started going directly to small local farms to purchase our meat, poultry, and dairy products. Before long, Lydia even convinced me to convert our property into an organic fruit and vegetable farm. Our four kids loved it because we added chickens, guinea fowl, and horses. Now we plant, water, weed, harvest, and can. And when we say grace, we mean it.

Besides changing the way I look at food, this transformation got me searching earnestly for a food-related book topic. That's when I came across Bill Marler. He's hard to miss if you get anywhere near food safety. After a couple of lengthy phone interviews, I visited Bill in Seattle in late June 2009. He picked me up at the ferry dock on Bainbridge Island in his red Volkswagen—license plate "ECOLI"—and took me to his home for our first face-to-face interview. It lasted two days! I'm serious. With some breaks for meals and sleep (I slept on an air mattress in his den), we covered everything from his childhood to his first marriage and subsequent divorce to the nuts and bolts of the Jack in the Box outbreak. He laughed about parts of his life and cried over others. I got goose bumps and I knew then and there that I had the right person to drive a narrative.

But getting Bill to cooperate wasn't enough. To truly portray the man who was the engine behind the Jack in the Box litigation, I needed his wife and children on board, too. I wanted an unvarnished look. That meant spending many hours in the Marler home—eating with them, going places with them, and being able to dig into their background. By the time I left Seattle after that initial visit, Bill's wife, Julie, had agreed to go along with the project.

It's fair to say that without the Benedict family and the Marler family, this book doesn't get written. Mine inspired me to write it. The Marlers gave me their trust and the access. For two years our families lived through the experience of writing a book. It was a journey. Along the way I came to admire and respect Bill and Julie. I'm honored to count them among my friends.

Still, it took the cooperation and trust of many additional players to make this story complete and compelling. Bob Nugent and Dave Theno opened my eyes to Jack in the Box's perspective. That's a side that's never been told. Yet it is vital to understanding the whole picture. I'm grateful to Bob and Dave for many, many hours of phone calls, interviews, and face time in San Diego. Both are as honest as they come.

Physicians Phil Tarr in St. Louis, Richard Siegler in Salt Lake City, and Glen Billman in San Diego, along with epidemiologist John Kobayashi in Seattle, furnished me with studies, reports, and statistics on *E. coli*. With these four medical experts as my guides, I felt like a journalist in medical school. Quite a club! All four submitted to interviews and many follow-up queries to ensure that I understood and properly reported the medical and microbiological aspects of the case.

The entire staff at the Marler Clark law firm bent over backward to assist me in digging through files, records, and reports. For weeks I set up shop in their offices to do research and conduct interviews. I'm particularly indebted to Peggy Paulson, Debbie Carr, Bruce Clark, and Patti Waller. Denis Stearns, in particular, was a machine when it came to producing key documents and exhibits. He also gave some mighty poignant and forthcoming interviews. Of all the people I came to admire along the journey, he's among the top of the list.

Mark Griffin at Keller Rohrback was an invaluable resource in providing me with court documents, pleadings, and checking billing records in an attempt to nail down key points in the legal time line.

A host of lawyers—Lynn Sarko, Chris Pence, George Kargianis, Simeon Osborn, Mike Watkins, Dick Krutch, Fred Gordon, Brad Keller—were all interviewed face-to-face and helped guide me through critical junctures of this complicated legal story. So did Judges Terrence Carroll and Lawrence Irving.

But all of this cooperation would have been for naught if Suzanne Kiner and Roni Austin hadn't agreed to relive the terrible ordeals of their daughters. My interviews with these two brave women were some of the most heart-wrenching sessions of my career. Tears streamed down my face when they'd cry and struggle to finish their sentences. As a parent, I could imagine the agony they went through. I'm grateful for their trust.

That covers those who were integral to helping me write the book. Then there's a remarkable team of people who worked on the book's publication. I'm a big believer in surrounding myself with extremely hardworking, talented people with a collaborative spirit. They are my colleagues, a true dream team.

Dorothea Halliday is a masterful editor with a relentless approach to detail and a great sense for tone and style. I think of her as Mrs. Thorough. Nobody does it better.

Attorney Chris Nolan is my legal editor; he puts me through the paces and always improves the read. His great judgment breeds trust and helps me sleep when the wind blows.

Beck Stvan is a superb graphic artist and he did a bang-up job designing the book jacket and overseeing art decisions. The guy just has serious skills and a great eye.

Andy Wolfe designed and produced a beautiful book and was a gem to work with on budgets, sales, and distribution. Aside from his great knowledge and experience as a publisher, his greatest asset is his can-do attitude. There aren't enough guys like him in the business.

Dee Dee De Bartlo and Gretchen Crary and the team at February Partners are the best publicists I've ever worked with—full of passion, creative ideas, and smarts. They work hard, smart, and fearlessly—my kind of people.

My personal assistant, Jeff Gasser, is a workhorse. He started in my office as an intern and quickly established himself as an irreplaceable colleague and trusted friend. He's going places, high and far.

My literary agent, Basil Kane, believed in this project from day one. His constant support is like his friendship—always there. He's been with me since my first book fifteen years ago. Ten books later we're soul mates.

I also get by with a little help from my friends. Armen Keteyian, Rob Wallace, B. J. Schecter, Mauro DiPreta, and Rick Wolff are friends who cause me to thank God for the extraordinary people he's placed in my path.

Of course, I finish where I started—with my love. So much of what I do and what I am starts and stops with Lydia. That goes for my writing, too. She was the inspiration for this book. She was my private editor and closest confidant throughout the process, reading early drafts and discussing direction and characterization. She's the smartest woman I know. Sometimes she leads me where I need to go. Sometimes she walks beside me. Other times she follows me. All I know is that her grace and beauty—inside and out—leave me breathless. Our children, Tennyson, Clancy, Maggie May, and Clara Belle, have an amazing mother, one who will make sure they eat safely and naturally.

SOURCE NOTES

The primary sources for this book are more than 250 interviews conducted by the author; written correspondence between the author and his sources; private photographs; and legal documents, medical records, and private papers in the form of notes, letters, and minutes made available to the author.

The secondary sources for this book include scientific studies, medical studies, government reports, court records, press releases, press reports, and other reference materials.

Many news organizations covered the Jack in the Box outbreak. I am particularly indebted to ABC News and CBS News for providing transcripts of news broadcasts and television news magazine coverage of the outbreak. I'm also indebted to the *Seattle Times*, particularly to Craig Ramsey, for furnishing me with dozens of print stories that tracked the outbreak. Also, Katie Salay, a research assistant at the U.S. Senate, was an invaluable resource in helping turn up hearing transcripts and government reports associated with those hearings.

Individual sources are included only in instances where I relied on another writer's original reporting, where I quoted heavily from a scientific or medical journal or from a newspaper article, or where my reporting produced conflicting results.

Chapter 3: Something Bad
Lee W. Riley, Robert S. Remis, et al., "Hemorrhagic Colitis Associated with a Rare *Escherichia Coli* Serotype," *New England Journal of Medicine* 38 (12): 681.

Chapter 8: An Awful Surprise
Susan Duerksen, "Girl, 6, Dies: Undercooked Meat Blamed," *San Diego Union Tribune*, January 20, 1993.

Chapter 11: Tell Me about *E. Coli*

Riley, Remis, et al., "Hemorrhagic Colitis"; Richard Siegler, "Long-term outcome and prognostic indicators in the hemolytic-uremic syndrome," *Journal of Pediatrics* 119 (5): 841–42.

Chapter 12: Testimony

"Jack in the Box's Worst Nightmare" (correction appended version), *New York Times*, February 6, 1993.

Chapter 14: No Miracles or Tragedies

Richard Siegler, "Recurrent Hemolytic-Uremic Syndrome Secondary to *Escherichia coli* O157:H7 Infection," *Experience and Reason*, available from the University of Utah Department of Pediatrics, Division of Nephrology, 50 North Medical Drive, Salt Lake City, Utah 84132 (ISSN 0031 4005).

Chapter 17: Nobody Blames You

Richard Martin, "Jack in the Box admits temperature rule error," *Nation Restaurant News*, March 1, 1993.

Chapter 19: Pickpocket

Michele Matassa Flores, "Jack-In-Box Agrees to Quit Asking for Releases from *E. coli* Victims," *Seattle Times*, March 5, 1993.

INDEX

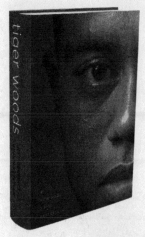
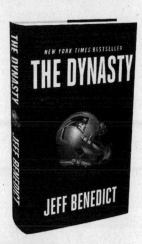
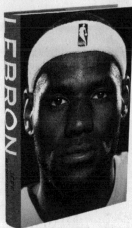